D1628517

RAPID REVIEW OF PACES
SECOND EDITION

WITHDRAWN FROM LIBRARY

BMA LIBRARY
BRITISH MEDICAL ASSOCIATION

An environmentally friendly book printed and bound in England
by www.printondemand-worldwide.com

Mixed Sources
Product group from well-managed
forests, and other controlled sources
www.fsc.org Cert no. TT-COC-002641
© 1996 Forest Stewardship Council
FSC

PEFC
PEFC/16-33-415

PEFC Certified
This product is
from sustainably
managed forests
and controlled
sources
www.pefc.org

This book is made entirely of chain-of-custody materials

BRITISH MEDICAL ASSOCIATION
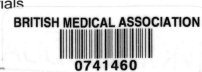
0741460

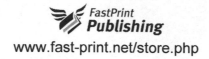

www.fast-print.net/store.php

RAPID REVIEW OF PACES
Copyright © Rashmi Kaushal, Sajini Wijetilleka & Sanjay Sharma 2014

ISBN: 978-178035-771-3

All rights reserved

No part of this book may be reproduced in any form by photocopying
or any electronic or mechanical means, including information storage
or retrieval systems, without permission in writing from both the
copyright owner and the publisher of the book.

The right of Rashmi Kaushal, Sajini Wijetilleka & Sanjay Sharma to be identified as
the authors of this work has been asserted by them in accordance with the Copyright,
Designs and Patents Act 1988 and any subsequent amendments thereto.

A catalogue record for this book is available from the British Library

First published 2011 by Fast-Print Publishing, Peterborough, England.

Table of Contents

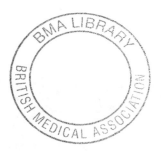

1 THE PACES EXAMINATION

The Practical Assessment of Clinical Examination Skills (PACES) examination consists of five clinical assessment 'Stations' where a selection of core clinical skills are tested by pairs of examiners using an objective marking system. Real patients and simulated or surrogate patients may appear, and clinical skills are tested in the context of standardised problems set in a variety of systems and settings. Examiners work in pairs to set the standard for each case, but mark each candidate without conferring. Each candidate is asked to demonstrate seven clinical skills, in eight patient encounters, and is assessed by a total of ten examiners.

Station 1	• Respiratory system examination	10 minutes
	• Abdominal system examination	10 minutes
Station 2	• History-taking skills	20 minutes
Station 3	• Cardiovascular system examination	10 minutes
	• Central nervous system examination	10 minutes
Station 4	• Communication skills and ethics	20 minutes
Station 5	• Integrated clinical assessment based on 2 observed clinical consultations	10 minutes
	- Brief clinical consultation 1	10 minutes
	- Brief clinical consultation 2	
	Total: 125 minutes (including 5 minutes between each station)	

1.1 Structure – the PACES carousel

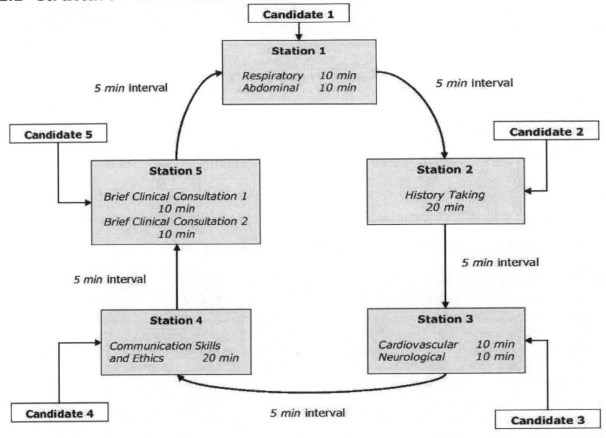

1.2 Details of each station

Stations 1 and 3 are also referred to as the Physical Examination Stations.
The emphasis in these stations is the demonstration of competence at:

- Clinical systems examination
- Eliciting with confidence, the clinical signs presented
- Presenting with accuracy, the clinical findings
- The ability to construct a differential diagnosis with investigation protocols
- Treating the patient with dignity, respect and professionalism at all times

The candidate will receive written instructions prior to each case examination

In the physical examination stations, 10 minutes are spent with each patient. 6 minutes are allowed for physical examination followed by 4 minutes for case presentation and questions from the examiners.

Each examiner will have a structured mark sheet for the case and every candidate will be examined by the same two examiners at each station.

Station 1: Abdominal and Respiratory

Example of written instructions to the candidate at the Respiratory station

This 39 year-old man is short of breath on exercise. Please examine his respiratory system, and tell the examiners what signs you find, and discuss your proposed management.

Example of written instructions to the candidate at the Abdominal station

This 55 year old lady has generalised itching and anorexia. Examine her abdominal system, present your findings and discuss your proposed management.

Station 2: History Taking

This is a 20 minute station. The candidate will have 5 minutes to read a letter written by a general practitioner prior to entering the examination room. 14 minutes are allocated to complete history taking. This is followed by a 1 minute reflection period for the candidate. The last 5 minutes are based on questions put forward by the examiners that are relevant to the case.

Both examiners will present and observing how the candidate conducts themselves in this station.

The history-taking skills station aims to assess the candidate's ability to gather information from the patient in the format of the traditional medical history and use this to construct a differential diagnosis and develop a management plan that is explained to the patient clearly.

The patient must be treated with dignity and respect at all times.

Example of written instructions given to the candidate at the History Taking station:

Patient details:	Mr Sajed Khan, a 54 year old gentleman.
Your role:	The doctor in a general medical outpatient clinic.
Presenting complaint:	Chest pain

Please read the referral letter below and prepare to conduct a history taking examination. You may wish to make notes on the paper provided.

When the bell sounds, enter the room. You have 14 minutes for your consultation with the patient, 1 minute to collect your thoughts and 5 minutes for discussion.

Dear Doctor,

Thank you for seeing this 54 year old year old gentleman who has been complaining of vague chest pains that occur most often in the evening. He was diagnosed with Hypertension, Diabetes and Dyslipidaemia 4 years ago and they are all well controlled on Ramipril, Metformin and Simvastatin.

He also has a history of acid reflux for which he takes Gaviscon.

His resting ECG has been normal as are his FBC and U&E's.

Many Thanks

Dr B Jones

Advice to the candidate:
- You will have 5 minutes to study this letter.
- Take the time to construct differentials and make a list of these on your notepad. This will enable you to cover the different causes for his symptoms and conclude the most likely cause for his symptoms as you take the history.
- You are expected to take a complete history which should follow the conventional format of:

PC:	Presenting Complaint
HPC:	History of presenting complaint
PMH:	Relevant past medical history
DH:	Drug history
FH:	Family history
SH:	Social history
A:	Allergies
GROS:	General review of symptoms.

Station 3: Cardiovascular and Neurological

Example of written instructions to the candidate at the Cardiac station

This 71 year-old man is thought to have a heart murmur. He is short of breath on exercise. Please examine his cardiovascular system, and tell the examiners which signs you find, and discuss your proposed management.

Example of written instructions to the candidate at the Neurology station

This 58 year-old man is troubled by weakness in his lower limbs. He is prone to falling. Please perform a neurological examination on his lower limbs, and tell the examiners which signs you find, and discuss your proposed management.

Station 4: Communication Skills and Ethics

This is a 20 minute station. The candidate will have 5 minutes to read the scenario.
14 minutes are allocated to complete the consultation. This is followed by a 1 minute reflection period for the candidate. The last 5 minutes are based on questions put forward by the examiners that are relevant to the case.

Both examiners will be present and observing how the candidate conducts themselves in this station.

This station will assess the candidate's ability to conduct an interview with the subject who is either a

- Patient
- Relative of patient or carer
- Surrogate such as a care worker, ward sister etc.

The candidate will guide the subject through a scenario which may involve explaining a diagnosis (in jargon-free terms so that the subject has understood what they are being told), or the emphasis may be on explaining a mistake, a missed diagnosis, dealing with a relative who is not coping or a patient who is reluctant to being admitted.

The candidate is expected to demonstrate honesty, respect and empathy during this consultation.

Example of written instructions given to the candidate at the Communication Skills and Ethics station:

Subject details	Mrs Gillian Miles Daughter of a patient on the ward
Your role	SHO on the ward
Problem	Explaining prognosis and care arrangements in a patient with terminal cancer.

Please read the scenario printed below.

You may wish to make notes on the paper provided. When the bell sounds, enter the room. You have 14 minutes for your consultation with the patient, 1 minute to collect your thoughts and 5 minutes for discussion. You may make notes if you wish.

Where relevant, assume that you have the patient's consent to discuss their condition with the relative/surrogate.

Role: You are the SHO on the ward. You have been asked to see the daughter of a patient of yours, Mr Frederick Jones. She lives abroad and only sees her father occasionally.

Scenario: Mr Jones is an elderly man with widespread metastatic carcinoma of the large bowel. He has been sent to A&E by his carers who feel that he has become too emaciated and weak to be looked after at home. He claims that he has had enough and does not further intervention. He has been seen by your consultant on the ward round and plans have been made for him to be seen by the palliative care team.

Your task is to discuss Mr Jones's prognosis with his daughter and suggest options about his on-going care.

Do not take the history again, except for details that will help in your discussion with the subject.

Station 5: Brief Clinical Consultation

The Brief Clinical Consultation station is used to assess a candidates approach to a clinical problem in an integrated and professional manner, using history taking, examination, and communication with a patient or a surrogate.

Each candidate will cover 2 cases lasting 10 minutes each.

Written instructions for each of the two cases, usually in the form of short notes or referral letters are given to the candidate during the five minute interval before this station.

Example 1: This 35 year old lady with arthritis complains of breathlessness. Please take a focussed history, examination and provide relevant feedback to the patient.

Example 2: This 58 year old man who is taking insulin has noticed that his vision has deteriorated. Please take a focused history, examination and provide relevant feedback to the patient.

Most cases will still be drawn from Endocrinology, Rheumatology, Dermatology and Ophthalmology. There will also be representation from Care Of the Elderly, e.g. Parkinson's, benign essential tremor and falls prevention.

Remember to read the explanatory referrals carefully, and identify the clinical problem(s) and develop a preliminary differential diagnosis based on the limited information available before seeing the patient, which will initially help guide the focused history.
- The history and examination should not be seen as separate components, where the history is followed by the examination. Both history and examination should be integrated. It is acceptable to take a history, then examine the patient, and then re-focus on the history.

The patient feedback is a vital component of this clinical encounter, which will carry a significant proportion of the marks.
- Explain the diagnosis or differential diagnoses using the techniques of checking and repetition, and avoid the use of jargon
- Relate these to the patient's symptoms to help him or her understand
- Explain your initial plans for further investigation and management, again avoiding jargon
- Address the patient's concerns

2 CLINICAL EXAMINATION

Although the format of the clinical part of the membership examination has changed, the basic requisite standard of clinical skill and acumen remains unchanged. There is an additional emphasis on the importance of effective observed history taking skills and communication which complements the clinical examination part of PACES.

By this stage it is likely that the majority of candidates will have developed their own styles and approaches to the clinical examination. However, the following serves as an outline of what this should encompass, and may be used by those who are yet to find a comfortably systematic technique as a template which they can refine. It should be noted that in no way should this be read as comprehensive, moreover as a guide covering the major systems overviews.

In addition to the basic algorithms of exam technique, there are accompanied pointers on how to interpret the elicited signs; something the candidate would be expected to be confident with. Finally at the end of the chapter is a section on overall exam tips.

Rule 1:   You never get a second chance to make a first impression
Make sure that you introduce yourself to the examiners and the patients. Smile to show that you are confident when dealing with patients.

Please try wherever possible to respect the Doctor- patient relationship. Introduce yourself as Doctor and never call the patient by the first name as it will detract from the formality of the situation. It may also irritate the old school examiners amongst us!

Rule 2:   If you don't look the part, you won't get the part!
Appearance is very important here: Please attend the examination dressed appropriately. I am often approached by female doctors who are not sure what to wear. I always suggest that a trouser suit, skirt suit or a dress are all appropriate as long as they look professional and are comfortable to allow for kneeling at the bedside. Ultimately, make sure that you look as attractive as you can without raising the patient's blood pressure.

For all candidates, it is essential that you arrive with clean-cut fingernails and preferably not smelling of cigarette smoke. Shoes must be polished and hair must be tidy.

For the male doctors, please make sure that you wear a suit and that it has been cleaned since you attended that wedding last summer. There is nothing more unsightly than mayonnaise stains on a tie or a suit collar!

Rule 3:   Bedside manners
Always ask the patient if you can examine them and give them clear instructions e.g. *"can you please show me your elbows"* or *"can you take deep breaths in and out through your mouth."* Please don't forget to leave the patient covered appropriately. Always thank the patient and then the examiners.

Rule 4:   Hygiene
With the advent of superbugs, many patients may have anxieties about contracting infection during the examination. Please be seen to be cleaning your hands between patients.

2.1 The Making of a Good Physician:

Many of you will be taking this examination for the first time. Some of you will be re-sitting for a second or third time. Whatever your situation, don't be disheartened. This examination will serve to make you a better Physician no matter how many attempts you make in order to succeed.

2.2 What is the Examiner Looking for?

The examiner needs to ascertain that you can be trusted to conduct a thorough clinical examination, interpret the signs and arrive at a competent clinical conclusion.

You must demonstrate understanding when moving from one system to another in order to demonstrate appropriate clinical signs e.g. cardiovascular system in Marfan's, or visual fields in acromegaly. You must maintain composure throughout, communicating your ease with patients and day to day examination of these systems.

2.3 General Approach to the Patient

Before you even begin to examine your patient, there are some basic do's and don'ts.

Make sure that you read the written instructions.
Instructions will usually be printed on an A4 sheet of paper under the patient's name. In some instances, the examiner may choose to repeat these instructions as an introduction to the case, e.g. "This is Mr Banes, he has been complaining of dizziness. Can you examine his cardiovascular system?" or "Mrs Hazel has lost weight and complains of breathlessness. Can you examine her respiratory system?"

Allow time for Inspection and start this as soon as you enter the room.
Whilst the examiner is introducing you to the patient, use that time to take in all the clues around in the room; is there a stick/crutch/cane? Does the patient wear glasses? Is he/she reading a book? If so, is the print size normal? Are there any adjuncts by the bed? If there is a sphygmomanometer or peak flow meter, it is likely that you will be expected to demonstrate competence in using it.

Examiner feedback:
One of the most irritating things examiners report is that they often feel that the candidate has not done what was asked of him/her. This may prove to be problematic as examiners are often unintentionally vague in giving instructions and written information has been introduced to overcome this. If despite having read the information outside on the door prior to entering, you are not clear, ask the examiner to repeat his/her instructions. The last thing you want to do is be unsure as to where to begin the examination of a patient complaining of fatigue! However, avoid mere ritualistic repetition, which often annoys examiners and also reduces the time available to you to examine the patient.

Introduction to the patient
ALWAYS introduce yourself to the patient. Your examiners may refer to you by your candidate number; however for the purposes of the examination, it is better to introduce yourself to the patient by your name. From the outset it is likely that this will make the patient feel less inhibited (even the 'professional' exam patients) and sounds better than "Hello. I am candidate number three hundred and twenty-two."

- As you approach the patient, keep your eyes open and look for any additional clues that may be more apparent as you come closer. Look at the patients face and make eye contact. Scan the face for obvious abnormalities such as a Bell's palsy, upper 7th nerve lesion, stigmata of scleroderma or chronic liver disease. Look out for skin rashes; nail changes, excoriations (suggestive of pruritus and a pointer to underlying chronic liver disease), any scars, splints (carpal tunnel syndrome or radial nerve palsy) and so forth. Assess the general state of the patient e.g. comfortable, cachexic, cyanosed, distressed, blind etc.

- If the patient is not in the ideal position for examination of the relevant system (e.g. semi-recumbent for cardiovascular examination and respiratory examinations, and flat for the abdominal examination) inform the examiner that you would like the patient re-positioned. It comes across better if you undertake this step spontaneously, after asking the patient. Do not assume that you have to examine the patient as you find them, if they are inappropriately positioned. Equally, however be ready to explain to the examiner why you are re-positioning the patient if he/she asks you (i.e. to discern the height of the jugular venous pulse in the cardiovascular examination and to relax the anterior abdominal wall musculature when examining the abdominal system). Remember that whilst you re-position the patient, you may have the only opportunity to INSPECT the back of the chest and other areas, where there may be additional clues as to the underlying diagnosis.

- Be GENTLE! When you do begin the examination always start by asking the patient if they have any PAIN anywhere. It would be foolish to offer a handshake to a patient when you introduce yourself if they have actively inflamed joints! The art of palpation really is an art; it has to be effective and, in experienced hands, looks graceful. Before taking this examination, you will need to have mastered this and practice will make perfect.

- After your examination is complete, finish by covering the patient if exposure has been required, and cordially THANK them. This courteous gesture is a very crucial part of the examination and has important significance to both the patient and the examiner, about your overall conduct. When you have done this, turn to the examiner and deliver your findings and offer a diagnosis, or differential diagnoses.

- Try not to keep turning or looking back at the patient whilst presenting your findings to the examiner! Examiners may find this irritating and interpret this as an uncertainty on your part. The presentation ideally has a beginning (general state of patient), middle (key findings) and an end (possible differential diagnoses).

- Use appropriate medical terminology **at all times**. In acromegaly avoid the word "big", the patients will be fed up with such pre-school observations which will be both insulting to the patient and reflective of your own ignorance. Use medical terminology like "prominent periorbital ridges", "enlarged extremities", "macroglossia" instead of big head, big nose, and big tongue.

- When you have finished offering your findings or diagnosis and have answered the examiners additional questions, finish this station by thanking the examiner before moving on. Again this is very courteous and can enhance the overall impression that the examiner has of you.

- When you do leave any particular station, it is absolutely crucial that you leave behind any questions or points in the previous examination that are still lingering in your mind. Every station in the PACES examination needs to be thought of independently. A common theme amongst candidates who don't do well in the examination is that they get 'hung-up' on their previous case/station and lose focus on the station at hand. Once you let this happen, it is difficult to then pick yourself up, something akin to the 'domino effect'.

2.4 Examination of the Cardiovascular System

It is unlikely that you will be asked directly to "Examine this patient's cardiovascular system". Ultimately however, that is what is expected at this station.

You must be able to perform the entire examination comprehensively. This therefore entails beginning the examination with general inspection, examination of the hands and finishing by assessing the functional status (signs of heart failure); remembering throughout, that you are not only trying to ellicit the signs, but also to give thought to the possible underlying causes.

The instructions given to you will aim to provide additional information and give clarity on what is to be expected from you.

Written instructions:
- This lady complains of breathlessness and palpitations. Examine the cardiovascular system.
- The 75 year old man presented with a chest pain and syncope. Examine his cardiovascular system
- This elderly lady presented with an acute episode of breathlessness. She was found to have a murmur. Examine the cardiovascular system.
- This patient has been referred by his GP for investigation of a heart murmur. Please examine and advise.

Ensure your hands are clean. Approach the patient from the right hand side and ensure that he is ideally positioned reclining at 45° and that he has removed any clothing to expose his chest neck and abdomen. You will have an opportunity for general inspection at this time.

2.4.1 Inspection – General

- **Young fit patient**: Make sure that you don't miss a VSD, corrected ASD, corrected Coarctation, corrected Fallot's or a dextrocardia.

- **Obvious syndromes** e.g. Down's syndrome or Turner's. Be prepared to comment on these findings, other systems involvement as well as what you find on cardiac examination. Add reference to these cases as per pages in the book.
    - **Marfan's Syndrome**: Tall stature, arachnodactyly, hypermobile joints, high arched palate, arm span exceeds height, possible pectus excavatum or scoliosis. Look for evidence of mitral valve prolapse or aortic regurgitation.
    - **Acromegaly**: Large doughy spade shaped sweaty hands, coarse facies, macroglossia, increased inter dental spacing, scars of carpal tunnel decompression. Look for cardiomegaly and displaced apex beat.
    - **Other Dysmorphic Syndromes:** William's, Noonan's. William's syndrome (short stature, pectus excavatum, clinodactyly – inward bend of little finger, flattened nasal bridge, prominent lips, skin that covers epicanthic folds, can be linked with aortic stenosis or pulmonary stenosis). Noonan's syndrome is an autosomal dominant syndrome associated with short stature, scoliosis, hypotonia, growth retardation, widely set eyes (hypertelorism), epicanthic folds and nystagmus, low set ears, pectus excavatum, short stature, pulmonary stenosis, ASD and HOCM.
    - **Ankylosing Spondylitis**: question mark posture (due to loss of lumbar lordosis, fixed kyphoscoliosis of the thoracic spine with compensatory

extension of the cervical spine, Look for aortic regurgitation seen in approximately 4% of patients.

- **Facial Nerve Palsy** – previous CVA, linked with patent foramen ovale/atrial myxoma.

2.4.2 Inspection – Specific

- **Malar flush**: A sign of pulmonary hypertension, seen with Mitral stenosis and Primary pulmonary hypertension
- **Breathlessness and Tachypnoea** (more than twenty breaths per minute)
- **Cyanosis**: A blue discolouration of the skin or mucosae. Peripheral cyanosis may be caused by reduced cardiac output e.g. mitral stenosis or shock or as a result of local vasoconstriction e.g. cold. It is best observed at the finger pulps and nail beds. Central cyanosis is caused right to left shunts of blood (with Eisenmenger's syndrome) by passing the lungs through a septal defect in the heart e.g. Fallot's tetralogy. It is best observed in the oral mucosa.
- **Pallor** : Anaemia causing heart failure or tachycardia
- **Clubbing**: A loss of nail bed angle, increased longitudinal and transverse curvature, perhaps a drumstick appearance. May be indicative of cyanotic congenital heart disease or subacute bacterial endocarditis
- **Splinter haemorrhages:** -vasculitis affecting the nail bed (infective endocarditis)
- **Janeway lesions**, painless palmar and plantar macules seen in infective endocarditis
- **Earlobe crease:** a visible earlobe crease is statistically correlated with coronary artery disease, especially in the Asian population
- **Visible neck pulsations**
  - **Corrigan's sign**: visible carotid pulsation, may be seen with harmonious head nodding (De Musset's sign) of aortic incompetence. Also seen in coarctation of the aorta
  - **Large *V* waves**: Occur in Tricuspid regurgitation, pulmonary hypertension and congestive cardiac failure
  - **Cannon waves (giant *A* waves)**: Occur as a result significant of shortening of the P-R interval such that the atria contract at the same time as the ventricles. They are seen in complete heart block, atrial flutter, single chamber ventricular pacing, nodal rhythm, ectopics and ventricular arrhythmias.

Jugular venous pulse: with the patient semi-prone assess the character of the waveform (canon *a* wave, *cv* waves (seen in time with the arterial pulse, hence the alternative name 'systolic'), and 'x' and 'y' descents (pericardial tamponade), as well as height above sternal angle. Frequently, the earlobe may be seen to oscillate, with tricuspid incompetence (very prominent *cv* waves).

- **Scars:** lateral thoracotomy (mitral valvotomy) scar may be missed under the left breast unless specifically sought for; midline sternotomy (heart transplant, valve replacement or bypass surgery: check vein graft sites), infraclavicular scar of inserted pacemaker. Don't miss the scars of an AV fistula in the ante-cubital fossa.
- **Oedema:** look down to ankles, expose if covered. Check for pitting; depress for 3 seconds and release finger. When examining posterior lung fields, check for presence of *sacral* oedema.
- **Clicks:** listen carefully for the audible clicks of a clean prosthetic heart valve. However, don't be fooled in to thinking that the audibility implies it is a metallic valve, as biological valves may also produce audible clicks.
- **Bruises:** evidence the patient may be taking warfarin. Some patients may wear an emergency warfarin bracelet.

2.4.3 Examination Routine for the Cardiovascular System:

Systematically begin peripherally, proceeding to the precordium, and then examining for signs of cardiac failure (unless asked specifically to do otherwise).

Radial pulse:

Determine the rate (count for 15 seconds), rhythm (sinus, irregular) and character (weak/bounding). Either the brachial or the carotid artery should be sought to determine whether a 'slow rising pulse' is present or not. To examine for a collapsing pulse, place the three middle fingers across the strongest brachial impulse and then slowly lift up the arm, after establishing whether the patient has any shoulder discomfort, above the level of the heart. Simultaneously feel the other radial pulse in order to note any radio-radio delay (pre-subclavian coarctation, cervical rib). At this stage decide the appropriateness of examining for radio-femoral delay, by simultaneously palpating for the femoral artery pulse. Patients who have had a Blalock-Taussig shunt for correction of Fallot's tetralogy or those who have had large vessel vasculitis, e.g. Takayasu's may have an absent/diminished radial pulse.

Blood Pressure:

It is easiest to measure the blood pressure at this stage, as there is a high chance that you may forget to do so later at the end of the exam when you may be flustered by an intervening examiner. Often it will suffice to say to the examine that you wish to take the blood pressure, as he/she in most cases will usher you along, yet credit you accordingly for requesting to do so. This is all the more important if a sphygmomanometer is place by the patient.

Carotid pulse:

Assess at this stage if not already at the brachial artery for the 'slow rising pulse' of aortic stenosis. Also take this opportunity to confirm Corrigan's sign (a strong upstroke, followed by a rapid down stroke, which is often seen as well as being palpable when present.

Apex beat:

Move swiftly to the precordial region and localise the apex beat, by starting out in the axilla and moving medially (showing the examiner that you are considering left ventricular enlargement). Be seen to be counting down the rib spaces with the other hand, keeping the localising hand still. By starting this far laterally, you may pick up the lateral thoracotomy scar should have missed it in earlier haste. Additionally, the apex beat may be present on the right hand side of the precordium, signifying dextrocardia. Determine the character of the apex beat (thrusting/heaving or tapping as in mitral stenosis), as this may help in determining the dominant pathology in patients with mixed valvular disease. Additionally by placing the flat of the hand over the line of the lower heart border and by placing the hand over the precordium (left parasternal area) you may be able to detect any palpable heaves (right ventricular hypertrophy) or thrills (palpable murmurs). You may wish to take this opportunity to confirm the presence of apical-radial delay (in atrial fibrillation) if an irregular rhythm had been detected earlier.

Auscultation:

Listen over the precordium for the systolic murmurs of valve stenosis and diastolic murmurs of incompetence, remember that manoeuvres designed to enhance these murmurs may be required to make them more pronounced. You must be seen to be simultaneously palpating the carotid or subclavian artery in order to confirm the timing of the murmurs, despite being able to immediately recognise the nature of the murmur.

Left sided murmurs are best heard in expiration and the right sided murmurs in inspiration. Listen with the *bell* of the stethoscope over the apex beat with the patient leant to the left side (mitral stenosis). It is easiest to hear the murmur of aortic incompetence by listening with the diaphragm of the stethoscope held over the left sternal edge, at the end of inspiration, with the patient leant forwards. It is easier to appreciate by noting the absence of silence, and should be sought if other peripheral signs are suggestive of the diagnosis. If a murmur is heard, it is useful to note whether it radiates; the pan-systolic murmur of mitral incompetence may radiate in to the axilla, whereas the ejection systolic murmur of aortic stenosis may radiate upwards to the neck arteries (making the distinction from carotid bruits difficult). In addition to any murmurs, an 'opening snap' (heard best in the left decubitus position and appears promptly after the second heart sound), or a third heart sound may be heard (young healthy, mitral incompetence, left ventricular failure). It is extremely difficult to detect a fourth heart sound and it is best not to spend too much time trying to pick one out!

- The murmur of a ventricular septal defect is pansystolic.
- Common diastolic murmurs are those of aortic incompetence, pulmonary stenosis and the Graham-Steel murmur in severe mitral stenosis.
- Artificial heart sounds may be heard, indicating the presence of metallic valves. A click before the first heart sounds indicates a mitral valve replacement; a click before the second heart sound indicates an aortic valve replacement.

Hepato-jugular reflex:

Moving briefly to the abdomen, inform the examiner that you would like to examine for hepatomegaly. If he/she allows you to proceed than confirm hepatomegaly (right ventricular failure) and also determine whether it is pulsatile (tricuspid incompetence). At this point you may wish to confirm patency within the venous circulation by pressing firmly on the liver and observing for a rise in the jugular venous pulse in the neck.

Lung bases:

Auscultate briefly over the lung bases for the presence of signs of left ventricular failure (functional assessment). Use this opportunity to look for sacral oedema.

Other:

After completing the physical examination thank the patient and turn to the examiner and present your findings, after offering to measure the blood pressure, if you haven't done so already, or perform urinalysis and fundoscopy (signs of hypertension).

Rapid Assessment List for Cardiac Examination:

- Visual survey
- Pulse (rate, rhythm, character, radio-femoral delay)
- JVP: ?elevated, *a* and *v* wave dissociation (heart block), giant v waves (cannon waves) (tricuspid regurgitation),
- Apex beat (visible, displaced, tapping, thrusting)
- Sternal heaves, palpable thrills
- Cardiac Auscultation
- Position: Aortic regurgitation is best heard with the patient sitting forwards in expiration, mitral stenosis is best heard with the patient in the left lateral position.
- Auscultate the carotids
- Check for sacral and ankle oedema
- Auscultate the lung bases
- Palpate the liver
- Check the blood pressure
- Observe the temperature chart and urine dipstick
- Mention fundoscopy

2.4.4 Common short cases in Cardiology tutorials:

2.4.4.1 Aortic stenosis
- Pulse is regular, and slow rising in character
- The venous pressure is not elevated.
- The apex beat may be only slightly displaced to the left of the midclavicular line and is palpable as a forceful sustained heave.
- There may be a systolic thrill palpable at the apex, in the aortic area and the carotid region.
- There is a harsh ejection systolic murmur in the aortic region radiating to the carotids.
- The systolic blood pressure is low normal with a narrow pulse pressure.

Points For Consideration:

What is the definition of aortic stenosis?
The definition of aortic stenosis is based upon the valvular area. The normal valvular area is ~ 3.0cm ^{2} Aortic stenosis is normally graded as mild, moderate or severe.
- Mild: Valve area > 1.5cm^2
- Moderate: Valve area > 1.0 to 1.5 cm^2
- Severe: Valve area <1.0cm^2
- Critical: Valvular area < 0.75cm^2

What Factors are associated with progression of stenosis?
The natural history of aortic stenosis begins with a prolonged asymptomatic period which is associated with minimal mortality. In some patients, a mild degree of stenosis can progress to a critical lesion within a few years. Progression is manifested by:
- A reduction in the valve area
- An increase in the transvalvular systolic pressure gradient.

Whether patients who are at high risk of rapid progression can be identified is controversial. Some factors, which are thought to be of significance, are:
- Aortic jet velocity
- Degree of valvular calcification
- Hypercholesterolemia
- Renal impairment
- Hypercalcemia

2.4.4.2 Aortic regurgitation
- The pulse is regular, of good volume and collapsing in nature.
- The venous pressure is not raised.
- The apex beat is often displaced to the anterior axillary line and below the 5th intercostal space.
- There is an early diastolic murmur audible at the left sternal edge which is loudest with the patient sitting forward in expiration.
- The systolic blood pressure is high with a wide pulse pressure.

2.4.4.3 Mixed aortic valve disease
- May have some/all features of both pathologies and the candidate must determine which lesion dominates. There may be a bisferiens pulse

- Determining the dominant lesion: a small volume pulse with a narrow pulse pressure favours AS; a large volume, collapsing pulse with a wide pulse pressure favours AR.

2.4.4.4 Mitral stenosis

- Malar flush: accompanying pulmonary hypertension
- JVP: systolic 'cv' waves if there is accompanying tricuspid regurgitation secondary to pulmonary hypertension
- Pulse: Atrial fibrillation (AF) or may have may ectopics
- Left Parasternal heave- accompanying right ventricle (RV) enlargement
- Apex: Tapping apex beat; palpable S1(palpate apex and carotid simultaneously to determine-sometimes difficult if in AF);
- Heart Sounds: Loud S1; opening snap (high pitched sound heard best with diaphragm after S2, at apex in left lateral decubitus position); Loud S2 if pulmonary hypertension present.
- Murmur: low pitched rumbling mid-diastolic heard best with bell over apex in left lateral decubitus position. Accentuated by exercise (increase in heart rate). May be an accompanying early diastolic murmur of pulmonary regurgitation murmur (Graham-Steel) if there is concomitant pulmonary hypertension.

Examiner Questions

ECG findings: The commonest ECG changes consist of abnormalities in the P waves.

They may be Bifid as a result of left atrial hypertrophy or Sharp as a result of right atrial hypertrophy when there is high pulmonary vascular resistance and when there will also be evidence of right ventricular hypertrophy.

Points For Consideration

What is the main differential diagnosis of this murmur?
The mid-diastolic murmur can be mimicked by flow through an atrial septal defect (ASD) but the presence of a widely, fixed second heart sound, together with the absence of a loud S1, a tapping apex beat and no opening snap in the latter distinguishes the two conditions

How can you judge the severity of mitral stenosis?
The shorter the time interval between S2 and the opening snap, the greater the severity. The longer the duration of the mid-diastolic murmur, the greater the clinical severity of stenosis.

What are the main Chest X-ray features seen in mitral stenosis?
- A straight left heart border
- Upper lobe diversion
- Horizontal left main bronchus

What are the indications for treatment in mitral stenosis?
A 'tight' stenosis ($\leq$ 1cm^2), the presence of pulmonary hypertension and/or recurrent thrombo-embolism despite anti-coagulation are all indications for repair. Nowadays surgical replacement of valve is the procedure of choice but is less frequently performed in the Western world, as Rheumatic heart disease, the leading cause, is less prevalent now than a hundred years ago. However, with the influx of migrants from poorer parts of the

world, this may change. Other procedures include: close mitral valvotomy (look for the scar under the left breast); open/closed commissurotomy (calcified valves are less pliant and consequently not suitable for this treatment option)

2.4.4.5 Mitral regurgitation
- Pulse may be normal or jerky (reduced ejection volume because of regurgitation in to left atrium
- Apex beat may be displaced (associated heart failure)
- Heart Sounds: soft S1; additional S3 often heard
- Murmur: most often pansystolic radiating to axilla but can be mid/late systolic (if regurgitation is due to dilated left ventricle (LV)). Easily distinguished from tricuspid regurgitation by increased intensity in expiration.

Points For Consideration

How can you judge the severity of regurgitation?
The presence of a dilated LV (displaced thrusting apex), features of left heart failure are indicators of increased severity. There are those who also say that the presence of an S3 indicates a worse prognosis.

What are the indications for treatment in mitral regurgitation?
Surgical repair is indicated when the LV ejection fraction drops to below 60%.

2.4.4.6 Mixed mitral valve disease
- May have some/all features of both pathologies and the candidate must determine which lesion dominates
- Determining the dominant lesion: AF favours MS rather than MR but the latter can also cause AF; loud S1and Tapping apex beat favours MS; soft S1 favours MR; the presence of S3 suggests that accompanying MS is not severe. Features of pulmonary hypertension (malar flush; loud P2; accompanying TR; Graham-Steel murmur) favours MS rather than MR

2.4.4.7 Heart failure
- Signs of fluid retention: elevated jugular venous pressure, lung crepitations, pitting lower limb oedema, tender hepatomegaly.
- Evidence of poor perfusion: cold, clammy skin, low blood pressure.
- Evidence of ventricular dysfunction: displaced left ventricular apex, right ventricular heavy, third or fourth heart sound, functional MR or TR and tachycardia.
- Ascertain the aetiology – atherosclerosis, valvular disease, hypertension, myopathy, severe anaemia or volume overload, e.g. AV shunt.

2.4.4.8 Ventricular Septal Defect
- Pulse: normal
- Left Parasternal heave (if there is RV enlargement)
- Heart sounds/murmurs: absence of the normal splitting of S2 suggests that the left and right ventricle pressures are equal; a loud, harsh pansystolic murmur at the left sternal edge should also be heard

This is usually a young fit-looking patient. There may be evidence of Down's syndrome or Turner's syndrome. The pulse is regular and the venous pressure is not raised. There is a left parasternal heave which may be accompanied by a systolic thrill. There is a pansystolic murmur at the lower left sternal edge which is also audible at the apex. If there is coexisting pulmonary hypertension there may be a loud pulmonary second sound. There may also be evidence of secondary pulmonary incompetence as evidenced by an early diastolic murmur.

Note to the candidate:
Most haemodynamically significant VSD's are often treated surgically shortly after diagnosis in childhood. Generally the smaller the defect, the greater the pressure between the two ventricles and hence the louder the murmur. If a defect has occurred in the membranous ventricular septum just below the aortic valve this may persist and be complicated by late onset aortic regurgitation which may require surgical correction. Such cases require long-term follow-up.

Points For Consideration
How do you distinguish mitral regurgitation from a VSD?
Both can give rise to a pan-systolic murmur, but the location of the maximum intensity of the murmur should point to the most likely origin (apex in the former, left sternal edge with the latter). Also the murmur in a VSD is more or a harsh characteristic compared to that heard in MR.

What is Eisenmenger's syndrome?
This is the reversal of flow through a shunt, resulting in cyanosis as the pressures from the right heart exceed those of the left heart. This is most often seen in the context of shunts through VSDs e.g. in Tetralogy of Fallot but can occur in any shunt situation. Clinical signs to mention are clubbing, peripheral cyanosis, a small pulse volume and those of pulmonary hypertension. Signs of pulmonary hypertension and right ventricular hypertrophy on palpation are a left parasternal heave and palpable pulmonary valve closure. Auscultation should reveal a loud second heart sound, right ventricular fourth sound, a pulmonary ejection click, the early diastolic murmur of pulmonary regurgitation and the pansystolic murmur of tricuspid regurgitation.

2.4.4.9 Coarctation of the aorta

This is an uncommon short case. The constriction is usually distal to the origin of the left subclavian artery. Examine for:
- Greater development of the upper extremities and thorax.
- Visual scapular collaterals
- Radio-femoral delay
- On occasion the left subclavian artery is involved and there may be asymmetrical radial pulses
- Palpate for a thrusting apex, evidence of left ventricular hypertrophy and listen for the systolic murmur of coarctation, both anteriorly and posteriorly over the left upper thorax. Listen for the aortic systolic and (rarely) diastolic murmurs from an associated bicuspid valve, which may be heard over the scapulae. Revise the complications and associations of this condition.

2.4.4.10 Corrected Fallot's tetralogy
This is a cyanotic congenital heart disorder which comprises four separate defects:
- Ventricular septal defect with reversal of the shunt (right-to-left)
- Right ventricular hypertrophy
- Pulmonary stenosis
- Aorta that overrides the VSD

- Evidence of a Blalock-Taussig shunt; mild cyanosis, thoracotomy scar, left radial pulse is not as prominent as the right and the arm on the side of the anastomosis may be smaller than the other arm.
- Patients who have not received a shunt may be clubbed, cyanosed, have a left parasternal heave with normal left ventricular impulse and an ejection systolic murmur heard in the pulmonary area.

2.4.4.11 Patent Ductus Arteriosus

The pulse may be collapsing in character and regular in rhythm. The venous pressure is not raised. The apex is displaced to the anterior axillary line and is thrusting in nature as a result of volume overload. A left parasternal heave may be suggestive of pulmonary hypertension. On auscultation there is a continuous machinery murmur audible in the second left intra-costal space near the sternal edge. There is systolic accentuation of this murmur.

Differential diagnosis:
Other causes of continuous murmurs:
1. Membranous ventricular septum defect complicated by aortic regurgitation.
2. Aortic regurgitation accompanying mitral regurgitation.

2.4.4.12 Mixed Aortic & Mitral Valve Disease:
- Most commonly mitral regurgitation together with aortic stenosis
- MR with mid/late systolic murmurs may mask the AS murmur
- If the apex beat is displaced, MR dominates

2.4.4.13 Mitral Valve Prolapse:
- Pulse: ectopics
- Apex: undisplaced, normal character
- Heart Sounds/murmurs: mid-systolic click with a mid-to-late systolic murmur, the duration of which is reduced by short squatting exercises and increased by standing from squatting or performing a Valsalva manoeuvre

Points For Consideration
Mitral valve prolapse is most prevalent in young females who tend to present with atypical chest pain or paroxysmal arrhythmias. It may be seen in the context of connective tissue disorders such as Marfan's syndrome, Ehlers-Danlos syndrome or pseudoxanthoma elasticum, all which can make the mitral valve leaflets "floppy".

2.4.4.14 Prosthetic Heart Valves:
- Most commonly Aortic or Mitral
- Tricuspid prosthesis are more common in intravenous drug abusers
- Metallic valves produce an audible 'click'; porcine and cadaveric do not.
- Look for operative scars and signs of anticoagulation (bruising).
- Heart sounds: Listen for the metallic S1 and/or S2. Often this easier to do by ear whilst palpating the carotid pulse to time onset. Complex metallic valves may have more than one metallic sound, making identification of the replaced valve difficult. Similarly, concomitant AF makes timing with diastole-systole difficult. Systolic murmurs are often heard and do not suggest dysfunction but diastolic murmurs always indicate malfunction.

Points For Consideration

What kinds of prosthetic valves are used in clinical practice?
- Biological: Homograft's (cadaveric) & Xenografts (porcine)
- Mechanical: Ball & Cage (Starr-Edwards) & Tilt (Bjork-Shiley)

What are the main complications with prosthetic valves?
- Thrombo-embolism
- Dysfunction (leaky valve, blockage, dehiscence)
- Haemolysis (microangiopathic, especially with mechanical valves)
- Bleeding from over anti-coagulation

2.5 Examination of the Respiratory System
2.5.1 Inspection – General

a) Pickwickian Syndrome: obese, somnolent, malar facies, audible wheeze
b) Systemic sclerosis: beaked nose, shiny tight skin over face, telangiectasiae (associated apical fibrosis)
c) Ankylosing spondylitis: kyphotic spine (associated apical fibrosis)
d) Rheumatoid arthritis: symmetrical destructive arthropathy of the hands
e) Horner's Syndrome: ptosis, miosis, enophthalmos, anhydrosis (may be suggestive of an apical carcinoma

2.5.2 Inspection – Specific

a) Cyanosis- are there additional features of superior vena caval obstruction (facial and upper limb oedema, dilated superficial thoracic veins and fixed dilatation of the neck veins)
b) Respiratory distress- use of accessory muscles, tachypnea, grunting, intercostal/subcostal recession
c) Thoracic cage- shape (barrel: with chronic obstructive disease), *deformity* (pectus excavatum/carinatum) and *movement* (is there loss of the normal bucket-handle movement?). Asymmetrical chest wall movement is suggestive of a reduction in lung volume (collapse, pneumothorax, fibrosis or reduction surgery)
d) Purse-lip breathing: seen in chronic airways obstruction (esp. Emphysema). Not necessarily a sign of distress, as is a means of increasing the intra-thoracic pressure to open collapsed bronchioles.
e) Added sounds- listen carefully during your inspection for the sounds of polyphonic (multiple) or monophonic (large single) wheeze that results from airway obstruction, particularly in expiration. Is the respiratory cycle of normal duration (inspiration longer than expiration)? Sounds of upper airway obstruction may also be evident (grunting, gurgling, noisy/heavy breathing)
f) Scars- look for postero-lateral thoracotomy scars (lobe-pneumonectomy/ plombage). Note also the presence of any signs of previous radiotherapy (burns, telangiectasia, limb lymphoedema, Indian ink marks (for field identification))
g) Clubbing - suppurative lung disease (abscess, bronchiectasis or empyema), fibrosing alveolitis (absent in up to 60%), bronchial carcinoma, mesothelioma

2.5.3 Examination Routine for the Respiratory System
Start with the hands and proceed to the chest systematically.

a) Hands- whilst confirming finger clubbing, have a quick feel of the pulse (bounding) and examine for the presence of a flapping tremor (both seen in CO2 retention). Is there any small muscle wasting (apical tumour)? Then quickly proceed to the
b) Trachea- establish the position of the trachea (midline or deviated) by attempting to place a finger either side of it whilst keeping the middle finger centrally upon the trachea.
c) Lymphadenopathy- examine the patients neck from the back and axillae from the front for the presence of any enlarged lymph nodes. If present determine their character (hard as in carcinoma, rubbery as in lymphoma or tender as is often the case in viral infection)
c) Apex beat- confirm position, as displacement will signify mediastinal shift (interpret in conjunction with tracheal position). The impulse may be difficult to feel in the hyper-inflated chest.
d) Expansion- confirm the findings from inspection by placing a hand either side of the sternum and observe any loss of chest wall expansion during inspiration.

Ensure that you have assessed the expansion of both upper and lower lobes bilaterally (this requires performing this manoeuvre twice; above and below the breast)

e) Percussion- start in the supraclavicular fossae, comparing the sides then move down to below the clavicles. In order to adequately assess the percussion note, you do not have to percuss over every rib space. It is only necessary to percuss over the area of the underlying lobes. This means that the same information can be got by percussing in three places as thirty, provided some knowledge of the superficial lung anatomy is known (remember to percuss in the axillary region to assess the middle lobe)

f) Tactile vocal fremitus or vocal resonance- it is adequate to do one or other. It may be more fluent to assess vocal resonance, as this can be done at the end of auscultation. Use the ulnar border of the hand for tactile vocal fremitus. Ask the patient to repeat "99". Is there any Aegophony?

g) Auscultation- comparing both sides continuously listen over the lobes, not forgetting the lung apices. Is expiration longer than inspiration (asthma)? Is there wheezing? Inspiratory crepitations/crackles should be timed for when they occur in the respiratory cycle, as this may be a pointer to the underlying pathology; early-bronchitis/), early to mid- bronchiectasis (may also extend in to expiration), mid to late- lung fibrosis (fine) or pulmonary oedema (fine/coarse). Bronchial breathing (listen over trachea for confirmation) may be heard in lobar pneumonia; the presence of a pleural rub (crunching sound during inspiration) signifies pleural inflammation (usually infection/uraemia)

h) Posterior chest wall- one you have completed examining the patient from the front, perform the same routine from behind, taking the opportunity to note any scars that may have been missed initially.

i) Complete the examination by examining the sputum pot and asking the patient to blow in to the peak flow metre.

Rapid Assessment List for Respiratory Examination:
• Visual survey
• Pulse (rate, rhythm, bounding character,)
• JVP: Systolic 'cv' waves with TR secondary to pulmonary hypertension
• Check for supraclavicular lymphadenopathy (from behind)
• Tracheal position/tug
• Apex beat (difficult to palpate in hyperinflation syndromes)
• Sternal heaves (Pulmonary hypertension)
• **From Front & Behind:**
• Percussion
• (Tactile vocal fremitus)
• Auscultation
• Vocal resonance
• Check for sacral and ankle oedema
• Check the sputum pot, peak flow chart (check technique if meter present)
• Observe the temperature chart

Instructions

1. This lady presents with progressive dyspnoea. Examine her respiratory system.
2. This 55-year-old non-smoker has developed progressive breathlessness over the past two years. Please examine his respiratory system to determine a cause.
3. This lady has recently presented with haemoptysis. Examine her respiratory system.

4.   In rare situations, if on the day of the examination the patient is frail or has an exacerbation of the lung disease the examiners may insist that you examine the patient from the front. Instructions of this nature are usually for the patient's benefit and the understanding on the examiner's part that a prolonged examination may exhaust the patient. It is not unusual in such insistences that you may then be asked to examine the patient's chest from the back.

Examination routine

Inspection	General appearance. Evidence of cachexia. Features of systemic sclerosis; does the patient appear Cushingoid or have lupus pernio; are there any inhalers at the bedside or an oxygen cylinder; is the patient breathless at rest or does the patient become breathless with little effort such as removing clothing or adjusting himself for examination. Is there any evidence of accessory muscle breathing suggestive of airways obstruction, pulmonary infusion or pneumothorax. Is there evidence of indrawing of the intercostal muscles or the supraclavicular fossae as a result of hyperinflation. Is the movement of the chest wall symmetrical. Are there are any thoracotomy or thoracoplasty scars or any evidence of radiotherapy y field markings, which are usually done in Indian ink. Are there any radiation burns on the chest? **Go back to the bedside equipment**. Do you want evidence of sputum pot, inhaler therapy, nebuliser therapy, temperature chart, peak flow chart?
Examination of the hands	Look for tremor or any evidence of carbon dioxide retention. It may be a fine tremor due to beta agonist therapy. Check for central cyanosis by examining the tongue and the buccal mucous membranes. Is there any evidence of clubbing or tar-stained fingers. Are there any changes in the small joints of the hands in keeping with rheumatoid arthritis or scleroderma. Examination of the hands will also highlight any peripheral cyanosis.
Pulse	
Trachea	Arrange photograph for examination of the trachea
Lymph nodes	Examine the cervical region and the axillae
Apex beats	From the end of the bed ask the patient to take a deep breath in and out. Observe for asymmetry or any reduced expansion suggestive of pathology. Photograph. Grip the chest and ask the patient to take a deep breath in and out again to assess expansion.
Percussion	Photograph.
Tactile vocal fremitus	Photograph.
Auscultation	
Examine the back	Repeat expansion, palpation, percussion, tactile vocal fremitus.
	Complete examination by checking for evidence of ankle oedema. Observe any bedside charts.

During the inspection, look for evidence of Horner's syndrome, or wasting of the small muscles of the hands. Look for any evidence of a previous BCG scar. If there is a peak expiratory flow bin by the bed then use it.

2.5.4 Common Cases in Respiratory Medicine
2.5.4.1 Pleural Effusion:
- Reduced ipsilateral lung expansion
- Contralateral tracheal deviation if effusion is very large
- Stony dull percussion note
- Reduced ipsilateral breath sounds/ tactile vocal fremitus/vocal resonance

Points For Consideration
How would you classify the common causes of a pleural effusion?
- Exudate (>30mg/dl protein): Bronchial cancer; pneumonia; drugs (methotrexate, nitrofurantoin), TB; Rheumatoid; SLE; mesothelioma; PE; metastasis
- Transudate (<30mg/dl protein): Nephrotic syndrome; Cardiac failure; hypothyroidism; Yellow-Nail syndrome; Meig's Syndrome (Ovarian fibroma)

2.5.4.2 Chronic Obstructive Pulmonary Disease:
- Inspection: Nicotine staining may be evident on fingers. Blue (bronchitis)/ Pink (emphysema); Accessory respiratory muscles; intercostals recession; tachypnea
- Tracheal tug (<3 finger space between suprasternal notch & Cricoid cartilage)
- Hyper-resonant percussion note
- Quiet breath sounds
- Crepitations/polyphonic wheeze

Points For Consideration

What are the usual precipitants of an exacerbation?
- Smoking (triggering bronchospasm)
- Infection (most commonly *H. Influenzae*, *S. Pneumoniae* or *M. catarrhalis*)
- Bronchoconstricting drugs
- Exercise

What features help distinguish emphysema from chronic bronchitis?
- Emphysema: pink (acyanotic), hyperinflated barrel shaped chest, tachypnea, purse-lip breathing; no pulmonary hypertension/cor pulmonale
- Chronic bronchitis: blue (cyanotic), minimal hyperinflation, dyspnoea, cor pulmonale, coarse crepitations.

What is the role of non-invasive ventilation?
This is now being used more and more frequently as a means of avoiding endotracheal assisted ventilation, from which it is often very difficult to wean patients with COAD off. It provides pressure support through a face mask and has been shown to be of benefit in those with hypercapnic hypoxia. It is sometimes not well tolerated as the mask needs to be tightly applied to the face.

2.5.4.3 Cryptogenic fibrosing alveolitis:
- Finger clubbing
- ± rheumatoid hands, scarring alopecia, Jaccoud's arthropathy, Raynaud's, signs of systemic sclerosis (beak-like nose with tight skin, calcinosis of finger tips), malar rash
- bibasal fine end-inspiratory crepitations

Points For Consideration

How commonly is finger clubbing seen in this condition?
Finger clubbing is only seen in approximately 40% of patients with cryptogenic fibrosis, therefore it's absence does not weigh against the diagnosis. Finger clubbing should raise awareness for other underlying lung lesions such as bronchiectasis, lung abscess or tumour.

What other conditions can mimic the findings of cryptogenic fibrosing alveolitis?
- Connective tissue disorders: SLE. Rheumatoid arthritis
- Radiotherapy
- Chemotherapy drugs e.g. methotrexate
- Inorganic dust related interstitial lung diseases e.g. asbestos
- Granulomatous disease: Sarcoid, tuberculosis, berylliosis

What is the treatment of this condition?
High-dose steroid therapy (60mg Prednisolone) should be commenced following diagnosis (often involving a high-resolution, thin slice CT of the thorax) and continued for 4 to 6 weeks. If this does not achieve remission, then immunosuppressant drugs such as azathioprine or cyclophosphamide should be considered.

2.5.4.4 Apical fibrosis:
- Possible ipsilateral tracheal deviation
- Reduced upper zone expansion
- Dull percussion note
- Fine Inspiratory crepitation's in upper zone

Points For Consideration

What are the causes of upper lobe fibrosis?
- Old tuberculosis
- Radiotherapy
- Ankylosing spondylitis
- Connective tissue disorders: anti-Jo-1 (dermatomyositis)
- Extrinsic allergic alveoloitis
- Massive pulmonary fibrosis from pneumoconiosis

What other features of old tuberculosis should be looked for?
Other features evident on clinical examination are scars from previous plombage therapy (ping-pong balls/sponges used to collapse the infected lobe to prevent aeration and spread of bacilli), previous lobectomy/pneumonectomy scars (look at back, and under axillae) and scars from phrenic nerve crush surgery.

Can the cause of apical fibrosis be distinguished?
- Look for the telangiectasiae associated with radiotherapy across the chest wall.
- Look at the hands and skin for Gottron's papules and Garrod's pads to determine if there is co-existent dermatomyositis.
- Ask the patient to stand, to see if the typical "question mark" posture of Ankylosing spondylitis is present.

2.5.4.5 Cor pulmonale:
- Cyanosis
- Respiratory distress
- Systolic waves in the JVP
- Malar flush
- Ankle & Sacral oedema
- Parasternal heave
- Loud P2 with a pan-systolic murmur heard best in inspiration at the sternal edge. A pulmonary regurgitant murmur may also be heard.

Points For Consideration

What is cor pulmonale and what are the common precipitants?
Cor pulmonale is the enlargement of the right ventricular that occurs as a consequent to raised pulmonary artery pressure (pulmonary hypertension) that occurs secondary to chronic lung disorders (e.g. COAD, bronchiectasis) or disorders of the pulmonary circulation (recurrent pulmonary emboli, primary pulmonary hypertension).

What are the ECG features of Cor pulmonale?
- 'P' pulmonale
- Right axis deviation
- Right ventricular hypertrophy

2.5.4.6 Lung Collapse
- Ipsilateral tracheal deviation
- Decreased ipsilateral expansion
- Dull ipsilateral percussion note
- Reduced ipsilateral breath sounds

Points For Consideration

What are the common causes of lung collapse?
- Iatrogenic (therapy for tuberculosis)
- Bronchial cancer (extrinsic compression)
- Bronchial adenoma (intrinsic occlusion)
- Lymphadenopathy
- Mucus plugs
- Foreign bodies (Right side more commoner than left, as Right main bronchus is more vertical than the left)

2.5.4.7 Pneumothorax:
- Contralateral tracheal deviation (if large, and under tension)
- Reduced ipsilateral expansion
- Hyper-resonant ipsilateral percussion note
- Reduced/absent ipsilateral breath sounds

<u>*Points For Consideration*</u>

What are the causes of a Pneumothorax?

Primary or spontaneous pneumothoraces tend to occur in tall, thin men, where they may be an underlying connective tissue disorder. Secondary pneumothorax occurs in the context of Asthma and bullous chronic lung diseases such as emphysema. They are also seen in cystic fibrosis and other causes of bronchiectasis. One should be alerted to the possibility of pneumothorax in any trauma patients with sudden respiratory distress and similarly in patients who are being invasive ventilated (barotrauma).

2.6 Examination of the Gastrointestinal System

2.6.1 Inspection - General

a) α_1-anti-trypsin deficiency: should be considered if signs of chronic airways disease are evident on inspection (barrel chest, purse-lips, respiratory distress)

b) Wilson's Disease: dystonic movements together with Kayser-Fleischer corneal rings (requires slit-lamp examination to detect)

2.6.2 Inspection - Specific

a) Skin- colour (jaundice, pallor, ashen grey (Haemochromatosis, Addison's Disease), pigmentation (telangiectasia, scratch marks of pruritus, spider naevi, hyper-pigmentation of palmar creases). Loss of secondary sexual hair may signify genital hypoplasia. Superficial venous dilatation may signify portal hypertension or inferior vena caval obstruction.

b) Hands- clubbing (chronic liver disease, inflammatory bowel disease), leukonychia (low protein state), koilonychias, beau's lines, tendon xanthomata (nephritic syndrome, PBC) Dupuytren's contracture, palmar erythema

c) Flapping tremor- a coarse flap (need to evaluate for 30s to safely rule out presence) may indicate decompensated chronic liver disease. A fine tremor may indicate ciclosporin treatment.

d) Scars - are there tattoos (would support viral hepatitis in the differential diagnosis)? Scratch marks would suggest pruritus (cholestasis). Inspect the antecubital fossae for the presence of an arterio-venous fistula (end stage renal disease; may be on renal replacement therapy/have been in the past). Look for scars in the iliac fossae and lumbar regions (nephrectomy and transplanted kidney)

e) Masses- is the entire abdomen enlarged (ascites) or are there identifiable masses within the abdomen (transplanted kidney). Ask the patient to lift only his/her shoulders of the bed to reduce any herniae that may be present. Don't forget to look at the umbilicus, where a superficial carcinomatous nodule may be present (Sister Mary Joseph's nodule). Note any gynaecomastia in the male breast. Are there any pulsatile masses? If so there expansility should be determined.

2.6.3 Examination Routine for the Gastrointestinal System

Ensure that the patient is ideally positioned and exposed (explain to the examiner that a limited exposure may be more appropriate)

a) Hands- confirm the findings on inspection, feeling in particular for the nodular contracture of Dupuytren's or any xanthoma at the elbow

b) Eyes- note any xanthelasma around the eyes. Any arcus (white rim) is often seen around the pupil in those aged 40 and above. Look for conjunctivae pallor (retract lower eyelid), and scleral icterus (retract upper eyelid).

c) Mouth- angular chelitis (iron deficiency), glossy red stomatitis (B_{12} deficiency or Kawasaki disease), ulcers within the oral cavity (Crohn's disease), telangiectasia (Hereditary haemorrhagic), pigmentation at the vermilliform border (Peutz-Jeghers), buccal hyper-pigmentation (Addison's disease)

d) Lymphadenopathy- briefly examine from the front for Virchow's node (left supraclavicular fossae). If enlarged nodes are present a more comprehensive examination may be required. Ideally sit the patient up. This will also enable you to look for nephrectomy scars on the lower back.

e) Distended abdominal wall veins- determine the direction of flow; away from the umbilicus (portal hypertension) and upwards from the groin in inferior vena cava obstruction.

f) Palpation- Start by establishing where, if anywhere, the patient is experiencing pain! If a pulsatile mass had been noted, determine if it is expansile (aneurysmal) by placing the fingers of both hands either side of the mass. Then palpate the abdomen initially lightly and then deeply, proceeding in a systematic manner starting in the right iliac fossa (be meticulous, as often candidates actually start in the lumbar region and don't actually examine the iliac fossae, thus missing the transplanted kidney). Work your way round covering all the quadrants and noting any masses or areas of tenderness. Once completed go on to specifically examine for hepato-splenomegaly as follows

g) Hepatomegaly- start by palpation in the right iliac fossa and move upward with the fingers of the right hand perpendicular to the costal margin, until you feel the liver edge rise and fall against your fingers with respiration. Determine that nature of the enlargement (smooth, hard, craggy). Establish that the mass is truly hepatic by attempting to get above it. Establish that the mass, if hepatic, is not just a downwardly displaced liver (COPD) by percussing downward from the ipsilateral nipple until dullness is detected. Then proceed to percuss over the liver to determine if the mass has a cystic nature (polycystic kidneys, liver, pancreas) and confirm the extent of enlargement.

h) Splenomegaly- starting in the right iliac fossa palpate and then percuss diagonally towards the left hypochondrium, feeling for the edge of an enlarged spleen (dullness). The notch should be confirmed and the extent of enlargement should be noted. Splenic enlargement is supported by the inability to get above or ballot the mass. Movement with respiration would be expected.

i) Kidneys- masses in either hypochondrial regions should be distinguished from kidneys; the latter being ballotable, fairly fixed, and possible to get above. The overlying percussion note may be resonant (bowel loops or cysts)

j) Percussion- percuss along the sagittal plane noting any areas of dullness (especially flanks); if detected ask the patient to roll to the opposite side, keeping your fingers firmly over the point of maximum dullness and after about 5-10 secs repeat percussion. Any shift in the dullness, is suggestive of displaced fluid (ascites).

k) Auscultation- listen for renal bruits, bowel sounds. You may also wish to map out the extent of organomegaly by performing the scratch test.

l) Conclude the examination by informing the examiner that you would like to examine the external genitalia, perform a digital examination of the rectum and perform a urine dipstick analysis.

Rapid Assessment List for Gastro Examination:
• Visual survey
• Inspect hands (pigmentation, contractures, liver flap)
• Lymphadenopathy (axilla, supraclavicular)
• Palpation of abdomen- general
• Palpation of abdomen- specific masses if identified above
• Palpation and percussion for hepatomegaly
• Palpation and percussion for splenomegaly
• Palpation for fluid thrill & percussion for shifting dullness
• Palpate for expansile & pulsatile mass of aortic aneurysm
• Auscultation for bowel sounds
• Examine for inguinal herniae (cough impulse)
• Examine for inguinal lymphadenopathy and external genitalia
• Check for ankle oedema
• Offer to complete by performing a rectal examination
• Observe the temperature chart and urine dipstick

2.6.4 Common cases in Gastroenterology

2.6.4.1 Hepatomegaly:
— Enlarged liver margin 3-4 finger breadths below costal margins.
— Is the liver - smooth & uniformly enlarged, hard and craggy with irregular edge or tender?
— ± signs of chronic liver disease (icterus, pigmentation, clubbing, palmar erythema, Dupuytren's contracture, spider naevae, scratch marks, gynaecomastia, scant body hair. If decompensated – jaundiced, ascites, purpura, flapping tremor and encephalopathic. Look for signs of portal hypertension – caput medusae)
— ± lymphadenopathy
— no visually obvious hyper-inflated lungs

Points For Consideration

What are the commonest causes of hepatomegaly?
— Liver cirrhosis +/- portal hypertension
— Metastatic deposits
— Right heart failure

Causes of:

Smooth Hepatomegaly: If signs of chronic liver disease are present:
— Cirrhosis of the liver with portal hypertension
— Hepatitis B and C
— Brucellosis
— Weil's disease
— CMV infection
— Pernicious anaemia
— Glycogen storage disorders
— Amyloidosis
— Budd-Chiari syndrome
— Amoebic abscess
— Emphysema
— Haemachromatosis
— Sarcoidosis

Smooth Hepatomegaly: If signs of chronic liver disease are not present:
— Primary tumours
— Lymphoproliferative disorders

Common Causes of Hard, Irregular Hepatomegaly
— Malignancy – primary or secondary
— Polycystic liver disease
— Macronodular cirrhosis
— Hydatid cysts (associated with eosinophilia) and Syphilis.

What are the Causes of Chronic Liver Disease?

- Alcohol
- Viral hepatitis (hep B is most common in health workers, hep C in IVDU/post-transfusion patients and hep D if previous hepatitis B virus infection).
- Auto-immune chronic active hepatitis
- Primary biliary cirrhosis
- Haemochromatosis (male, slate-grey pigmentation)
- Cryptogenic
- Cardiac failure
- Constrictive Pericarditis
- Budd-Chiari syndrome – develops acutely, no cutaneous features of liver disease and the liver is smoothly enlarged and tender. Risk factors – thrombogenic disorders, OCP use.
- Biliary cholestasis
- Toxins and drugs (methyldopa, methotrexate, isoniazid, amiodarone, aspirin, phenytoin, propylthiouracil, sulphonamides)
- Wilson's disease (Kaiser-Fleischer Rings, dystonic movements, tremor, rigidity, dysarthria)
- Alpha-one antitrypsin deficiency (evidence of emphysema)
- Other metabolic causes – galactosemia, type IV glycogenosis

What is the differential diagnosis of a mass in the right upper quadrant of the abdomen?
- Enlarged gallbladder (cholangiocarcinoma, stone on cystic duct, obstruction at porta hepatis)
- Nephromegaly
- Enlarged lymph nodes
- Collection in Pouch of Rutherford-Morrison (para-colic gutter)
- Adrenal tumour
- Colonic tumour of the hepatic flexure
- Dilated bowel loops

How can you differentiate between nephromegaly and hepatomegaly?
The liver moves downward with inspiration, the kidney being retroperitoneal moves very little with respiration. The kidney can be bi-manually ballotted, the liver cannot. The percussion note overlying the liver is usually dull (unless it is cystically enlarged), whereas as it is usually resonant over the kidney due to super imposition of bowel loops.

2.6.4.2 Splenomegaly:
- Comment on enlargement below the left costal margin
- Characterise spleen – cannot get above mass, percussion note = dull.
- ± anaemia
- ± lymphadenopathy
- enlarged splenic edge to beyond the umbilicus, with a palpable notch

Points For Consideration

What is the normal position of the spleen?
In the absence of disease the spleen is usually impalpable, as it lies along the plane of the 9-11th ribs below the left costal margin.

What are the causes of splenomegaly?
- Chronic myeloid leukaemia/myeloproliferative disorders (PRV, myelofibrosis)
- Hodgkin's lymphoma/ other lymphoproliferative disorders
- Portal hypertension
- Congestive cardiac failure
- Malaria/leishmaniasis, hepatitis, bacterial endocarditis, salmonella.
- Hereditary spherocytosis
- Felty's syndrome (leg ulcers, neutropenia, rheumatoid arthritis)

How can you differentiate clinically between nephromegaly and splenomegaly?
The kidney moves very little with inspiration, whereas the spleen moves towards the right iliac fossa. The spleen has a palpable notch along its' medial border. The kidney is bi-manually ballotable, the spleen is not. The spleen usually has a dull percussion note over it (unless it contains a large cyst), the kidney may have either a dull or more frequently a resonant percussion note over it.

What is the cause of chronic myeloid leukaemia?
Chronic myeloid leukaemia is an abnormal proliferation of mature granulocyte precursors in the bone marrow that arises as a result of genetic aberration in these cells. This results in the constitutive activation of the tyrosine kinase receptor in these cells that occurs following juxtaposing of the 'abl' gene with y the 'bcr' inducer gene after a translocation mutation on chromosome 22. Karyotype analysis reveals the pathognomic 'Philadelphia chromosome' which is present in 95% of patients (and confers a better prognosis). The condition is now treatable with a metabolic receptor blocking agent, as well as bone marrow transplantation, both of which offer a good prognosis.

What is Felty's Syndrome?
Felty's syndrome is a rare complication of Rheumatoid arthritis characterised by neutropaenia, leg ulcers and splenomegaly. This results in recurrent Gram positive infections, which are the usual cause of death.

What are the indications for Splenectomy?
Splenectomy is indicated when splenomegaly results in hypersplenism (over destruction of all blood celll types) that is recalcitrant. This is most often the case in hereditary spherocytosis, Gaucher's disease, auto-immune haemolytic anaemia and sometimes is in thalassemia. Other indications include symptoms of mass effect from massive splenomegaly.

What measures should be taken post-splenectomy?
Patients should be informed pre-operatively of the lifelong risk of simple infections and the need to take prophylactic antibiotic cover with oral penicillin and the need for immunisation against the common pneumococcal pathogens (pneumovax).

2.6.4.3 Ascites:
- Abdominal distension
- Fluid thrill (if large volume of ascitic fluid)
- Shifting dullness

Points For Consideration

What are the causes of ascites?
The causes can be listed by virtue of the protein content of ascitic fluid:

- Transudate (<25g/l): congestive cardiac failure, constrictive pericarditis, Meig's syndrome, hypoproteinameic states (nephrotic syndrome)
- Exudate (>25g/l): cirrhosis (portal hypertension), peritonitis, malignancy, tuberculosis
- Chylous ascites

Question: How would you investigate ascites?
Send sample for diagnostic paracentesis – treat for SBP if more than 250 white cells/cm^3. Send sample for albumin, LDH, glucose and protein. Ascertain if ascites is exudative or transudative by calculating serum albumin-ascites gradient (SAAG).

High gradient

A high gradient (> 1.1 g/dL) indicates the ascites is due to portal hypertension with 97% accuracy. This is due to increased hydrostatic pressure within the blood vessels of the hepatic portal system, which in turn forces water into the peritoneal cavity but leaves proteins such as albumin within the vasculature.

Important causes of high SAAG ascites (> 1.1 g/dL) include:

- high protein (> 2.5): heart failure, Budd Chiari syndrome
- low protein (< 2.5): cirrhosis of the liver[3], nephrotic syndrome

Low gradient

A low gradient (< 1.1 g/dL) indicates causes of ascites not associated with increased portal pressure such as tuberculosis, pancreatitis, nephrotic syndrome and various types of peritoneal cancer.

What is portal hypertension?
Portal hypertension is usually a sequale of cirrhotic liver disease, whereby the pressure in the portal vein is abnormally raised. This results in splenomegaly and ascites as the pressure in the tributary veins is raised because of back pressure. Other causes can include 'post-hepatic' obstruction from hepatic vein thrombosis (Budd-Chiari syndrome) or extrinsic compression at the porta hepatis from lymph nodes ('pre-hepatic').

How would you manage a patient with ascites?
- Strict sodium and fluid restriction (the latter especially if sodium is very low)
- Diuretic therapy, often requiring combination therapy of a loop diuretic such as Frusemide, together with a potassium sparing diuretic such as Spironolactone. If this fails bumetanide or metolozone should be considered.
- The above should be monitored with hourly urine output and daily weight charts.
- Repeated paracentesis should be avoided as the ascites just re-accumulates and only increases the risk of peritonitis which can decompensate the underlying liver disease
- Trans-jugular intrahepatic porto-systemic shunting creates a side-to-side anastomosis between the portal and hepatic veins in order to relieve the high venous pressures.

2.6.4.4 Transplanted kidney:
- Cushingoid appearance
- Bruising
- Cateracts
- Hirsuitism (tacrolimus)
- Basal cell carcinomas
- Tremor (ciclosporin)
- Gum hypertrophy (ciclosporin)
- Signs of previous renal replacement therapy – AV fistulae, tunnelled lines.
- Arteriovenous fistulae (wrist/arm)
- Fullness in flanks
- Swelling under scar in right iliac fossa
- Masses may be palpable in flanks (if polycystic kidneys)
- Midline laparotomy scar/ posterolateral subscostal scar (nephrectomy)
- Palpable, non-mobile notched mass in left/right iliac fossa

Points For Consideration

What are the commonest causes of end-stage renal failure?
- Diabetes mellitus
- Hypertensive renal disease
- IgA nephropathy (glomerulonephritis)
- Polycystic kidney disease
- Bilateral chronic pyelonephritis

What measures are taken to ensure graft survival in transplant patients?
Pre-operatively, assiduous immunological matching is performed in unrelated donor-recipient pairs including HLA and blood group matching. Blood transfusions are avoided and any co-morbidity minimised e.g. CABG performed for chronic angina prior to renal transplantation. Post-operatively, immunotherapy is started and continued long term. The standard regimen includes: prednisolone, azathioprine and cyclosporine, which requires dose monitoring and adjustment.

What types of graft rejection do you know of?
- Hyperacute: preformed antibody mediated (ABO mismatch)
- Acute: mixed humoral and cellular response; may respond to high dose methyl prednisolone and/or anti-lymphocyte antibodies (OKT3)
- Chronic: cell mediated inflammatory response resulting in interstitial fibrosis, tubular obliteration; is irreversible and treatment is thus supportive, until a further graft becomes available.

Which diseases often lead to renal transplantation with poor outcomes?
- Haemolytic Uraemic Syndrome
- Sickle cell anaemia
- Systemic sclerosis
- Focal glomerulosclerosis
- Oxalosis
- Cystinosis
- Fabry's disease

2.6.4.5 Polycystic kidneys:

- Arteriovenous fistulae at wrist/forearm
- Bi/unilateral ballotable mass(es) in loin regions, with little or no movement with respiration and an overlying hyper-resonant percussion note.
- Transplanted kidney in right/left iliac fossa

Points For Consideration

Which other organs are affected in polycystic kidney disease?
Cysts may develop in the liver, pancreas, ovaries, spleen and the brain as well as the kidneys. Non-cystic manifestations include an increased predisposition to cerebral aneurysm formation and mitral valve prolapse. One kidney may be more affected than the other, giving the impression of a unilaterally enlarged kidney.

What is the cause of polycystic kidney disease?
In adults there is a genetic linkage to chromosome 16 to the PKD locus, and condition is inherited in an autosomal dominant manner. In children there is a linkage to chromosome 4, and the trait is inherited in an autosomal recessive manner.

How do adults generally present with polycystic kidney disease?
- Pain
- Haematuria
- Recurrent urinary tract infections
- Sensation of a mass
- Family history

Other causes of Bilateral Nephromegaly
- Bilateral hydronephrosis
- Amyloidosis
- Tuberous Sclerosis
- Von Hippel Lindau disease

2.6.4.6 Crohn's Disease
- Chronically swollen lips (granulomatous infiltration)
- Mouth Ulcers
- Multiple laparotomy scars – suggesting a chronic, relapsing abdominal condition which has led to crises requiring surgical intervention on several occasions.
- Abdominal fistula formation
- Dusky blue discoloration of the perianal skin
- Oedmatous skin tags, fissuring, ulceration and fistula formation

Other Features of Crohn's:
- Slim patient
- Anaemia
- Clubbing
- Erythema Nodosum
- Pyoderma gangrenosum
- Uveitis
- Pedal oedema
- Right Iliac Fossa Mass
- Arthropathy (rheumatoid pattern)
- Ankylosing spondylitis

Treatment
Steroids, immunosuppressants, anti-TNF alpha antibodies, surgery

Other causes of Anal Fistulae
- Simple fistula from an abscess of an anal gland
- TB
- Ulcerative Colitis
- Carcinoma of the Rectum

2.6.4.7 Haemochromatosis
- Thin patient with slate-grey pigmentation
- Decreased body hair and gynaecomastia +/- (and testicular atrophy – iron deposition affecting hypothalamic-pituitary function).
- Liver is enlarged at x cm (in 95% of patients; splenomegaly is present in 50%).

Other Features which may be present:
- Diabetes Mellitus
- Arthropathy (pseudogout)
- Cardiac involvement – large heart, dysrhythmias
- Hepatocellular carcinoma
- Testicular atrophy, gynaecomastia
- Addison's disease, hypothyroidism and hypoparathyroidism are extremely rare.

Facts about Haemochromatosis
- Autosomal Recessive inheritance
- Males > females
- Associated with HLA A3
- Gene responsible is located on the short arm of chromosome 6.
- Homozygous inheritance is responsible for 90% of cases in Northern Europe.
- Diagnosis is with serum ferritin levels, serum iron levels, HFE gene screening and liver biopsy.
- There may be a role for serial MRI of the liver.

Treatment
- Weekly phlebotomy – until haemoglobin is below 11g/dl; then maintenance phlebotomy to keep serum iron and ferritin in low end of the normal range
- When phlebotomy is initiated before cirrhosis develops, survival is normal.
- If anaemia and hypoproteinaemia are present then desferrioxamine is a better treatment. Concurrent ascorbic acid administration improves iron excretion.

2.6.4.8 Nephrotic Syndrome

There is *extensive oedema* affecting the ankles, lower legs and peri-orbital tissues of this patient. The skin is pale. There may be *white bands* across the nails (from chronic hypoalbuminaemia). There may be *bilateral pleural effusions and ascites.* (The patient may be hypertensive with tendon xanthomata to indicate hyperlipidaemia).

Commonest Causes

Glomerulonephritis (usually minimal change in children, membranous in adults)

The glomerulonephritides can be divided as follows:

1. Minimal change disease can be primary (idiopathic) or secondary to diabetes, lymphoma, carcinoma, AIDS or IgA nephropathy.

2. Focal and segmental glomerulosclerosis can be primary or secondary to infection (HIV), drugs (NSAIDS, opiates, analgesic abuse), diabetes, hypertension, Alport's, sickle cell disease, cystinosis and sarcoidosis.

3. Membranous glomerulonephritis. Primary. Secondary to infection (hepatitis B and C, malaria, schistosomiasis), connective tissue disorders (SLE, mixed connective tissue disease, dermatomyositis and Sjogren's syndrome), neoplastic (lung, colon, stomach, breast and lymphoma), drugs (gold, mercury, pencillamine) and familial in sickle cell disease.

4. Mesangiocapillary glomerulonephritis (primary idiopathic), secondary to SLE, cryoglobulinaemia, scleroderma, light and heavy chain disease.

5. Fibrillary glomerulonephritis – amyloidosis, multiple myeloma, cryoglobulinaemia, lupus nephritis. Malaria.

What are the investigations for Nephrotic Syndrome?
   - Urine microscopy
   - Urine protein selectivity
   - Creatinine clearance
   - Specific assays for causal diseases
   - Renal biopsy

What are the complications of Nephrotic Syndrome?
   - Thrombosis, Malnutrition
   - Atheroma and ischaemic heart disease
   - Infection

What are the Treatments for Nephrotic Syndrome?
   - Reduce dietary salt and lipid intake
   - Lipid lowering agents
   - Antihypertensives
   - Corticosteroids for certain types of glomerulonephritis
   - Steroid-sparing agents if required after this
   - Prolonged anticoagulation is required if recurrent episodes occur.

2.6.4.9 Carcinoid Syndrome
   - Cutaneous flushing
   - Facial telangiectasiae
   - Liver is palpable x cm below the right costal margin.
   - Liver edge is ir/regular.
   - History of flushing and diarrhoea

Other features of Carcinoid Syndrome
- Right sided valvular lesions due to 5HT induced endocardial fibrosis (pulmonary stenosis, tricuspid incompetence).
- Peritoneal and retroperitoneal fibrosis.
- Bronchoconstriction (20% of patients experience wheezing)
- Abdominal pain, weight loss and cachexia
- Diagnosed with very high urinary 5-HIAA levels
- Treated with somatostatin analogues, cyproheptadine and leucocyte interferon. Surgical debulking may also be required.

What are the ectopic humoral syndromes in histological carcinoid tumours?
- Cushing's syndrome (ACTH in bronchial carcinoid)
- Dilutional hyponatraemia (ADH in bronchial carcinoid)
- Gynaecomastia (HCG in gastric carcinoid)
- Acromegaly (GHRH in foregut carcinoid)
- Hypoglycaemia (insulin in pancreatic carcinoid)

Polycythaemia Rubra Vera
- Facial plethora
- Dusky cyanotic face and mucous membranes.
- Ecchymoses and scratch marks (from pruritus).
- Conjunctival engorgement.
- Splenomegaly.
- Perform fundoscopy and look for dilated retinal veins
- Check blood pressure.

Question: What are the diagnostic criteria for primary polycythaemia?
- Raised red cell mass, white cell and platelet count
- Raised Hb and Hct.
- Reduced MCV suggestive of iron deficiency erythropoesis
- Presence of JAK-2 mutation
- Exclusion of secondary causes of polycythaemia

Question: What are the diagnostic criteria for secondary polycythaemia?

Appropriate EPO production:
- Arterial hypoxaemia – COPD, right to left shunt, obesity hypoventilation syndrome
- Abnormal release of oxygen from Hb – congenitally reduced red cell 2,3 –DPG, smoking
- Interference with tissue oxygen metabolism – cobalt poisoning

Inappropriate EPO production:
Neoplasms- renal, adrenal, hepatocellular, ovarian, cerebellar, haemangioblastoma, phaeochromocytoma.
Non-neoplastic renal disease –such as cysts and hydronephrosis.

2.6.4.10   Generalised lymphadenopathy

Generalised lymphadenopathy with/without x cm *splenomegaly/hepatosplenomegaly.*
The most likely causes are *lymphoreticular disorders* (Hodgkin's or non-Hodgkin's lymphoma) or *chronic lymphocytic leukaemia.*

Other causes
- Infectious mononucleosis
- Sarcoidosis
- Tuberculosis
- Cytomegalovirus
- Thyrotoxicosis
- Retroviral disease

Diagnosis and Staging of Non-Hodgkin's disease – use WHO/Real classification
- Lymph node biopsy
- CT Chest/Abdomen/Pelvis
- Bone marrow aspirate and trephine
- MRI head in certain subtypes where CNS involvement is common.

2.6.4.11   Single Palpable Kidney
- Mass (describe consistency, edges, size) on the right/left side of the abdomen in the mid-zone.
- Bimanually ballotable and the percussion note is resonant over it. (Examine for signs of uraemia/previous dialysis).

Causes
- Polycystic kidney disease with only one kidney palpable
- Carcinoma – renal cell carcinoma accounts for 2% of adult malignancies, increased risk with smoking. Spreads to abdominal lymph nodes; distant metastases common in lung and bone. Haematuria is the most common presenting symptom. Treatment is with nephrectomy and immunotherapy (IFN alpha and IL-2).
- Hydronephrosis
- Hypertrophy of single functioning kidney – may predispose to proteinuria, hypertension and glomerular sclerosis

Case 11: Primary Biliary Cirrhosis
- Icteric and has pigmented skin
- Excoriated skin due to scratching.
- Clubbed fingernails and xanthalasma.
- Hepatomegaly and x cm splenomegaly.
- Ascites and pedal oedema.

Question: Which Investigations can be used to diagnose PBC?
- HLA phenotypes B8 and C4B2
- Anti-mitochondrial antibody positive in 95%
- Anti-Smooth muscle antibody positive in 50%
- Anti-nuclear factor positive in 20%
- Liver biopsy: stain for copper

Question: What are the treatments for PBC?
- Pencillamine – to chelate copper
- Immunosuppressants

- Anti-fibrotics, e.g. colchicine
- Ursodeoxycholic acid
- Supplementation of fat-soluble vitamins
- Cholestyramine
- Physiological intervention – bile diversion, haemoperfusion, charcoal column perfusion, plasmapheresis may be helpful in refractory cases.

<u>Question: What is this patient at risk of?</u>
- Bleeding oesophageal varices
- Malabsorption
- Osteomalacia

Question: Which conditions are associated with PBC?
Sjogren's, systemic sclerosis, CREST, rheumatoid arthritis, Hashimoto's thyroiditis, renal tubular acidosis, coeliac disease, dermatomyositis.

2.6.4.12 Abdominal Masses
<u>Causes of a Right Iliac Fossa Mass</u>
1. Ileocaecal TB

2. Carcinoma of the caecum

3. Amoebic abscess

4. Lymphoma

5. Appendicular abscess

6. Neoplasm of the ovary

7. Ileal carcinoid

<u>Causes of a Left Iliac Fossa Mass</u>
1. Carcinoma of the colon

2. Left ovary neoplasm

3. Faeces

4. Amoebic abscess

<u>Causes of a Left Upper Quadrant Mass</u>
1. Carcinoma of the colon

2. Retroperitoneal sarcoma

3. Lymphoma

4. Diverticular abscess

<u>Causes of an Epigastric Mass</u>
1. Carcinoma of the pancreas

2. Carcinoma of the stomach

3. Lymphoma

<u>Causes of a Pulsatile Mass</u>
    Aneurysm of the abdominal aorta (ensure you listen for bruits)

2.7 Examination of the Neurological System

Often thought of as the most difficult aspect of the examination, the neurological examination is relatively simple to perform. The relative difficulty lies in the interpretation of the findings. Consequently, this weakness can be overcome if the neurological case is approached in a systematic manner by performing a meticulous examination, in order to determine first of all, 'where the lesion/pathology is' and then by suggesting 'what could have caused the lesion'. This analytical approach is of particular use in problems in the peripheral nervous system where there is considerable overlap between the sensory and motor systems (see algorithm). Armed with this basic means of assessment and the recognition of the specific patterns of neurological dysfunction (see below), you should be able to display a fairly comprehensive performance during the examination.

2.7.1 Inspection – General
a) Myotonic dystrophy- frontal balding, fatigued myotonic facies, ptosis
b) Myasthenia gravis- female, bilateral ptosis, lid fatiguability
c) Muscular dystrophy- wheelchair, bilateral calf enlargement (pseudohypertrophy)

2.7.2 Inspection – Specific
a) Gait- observe how the patient walks; stamping (dorsal column loss), foot dragging (foot drop-CVA, S_1 root, peripheral neuritis), broad-base (cerebellar), spastic/circumducting (cord paresis), festinant (Parkinson's disease), high stepping (peripheral neuropathy). The gait abnormality may be exacerbated by asking the patient to heel-toe walk, walk on the toes or heels or by asking the patient to walk a few steps with their eyes shut (sensory ataxia)
b) Muscle bulk- look at all the muscle groups; note any atrophy or dystrophy and whether this is generalised (systemic cause) or focal (localised cause), proximal (muscle disease) or distal (conduction problem-peripheral nerve/root).
c) Fasciculations- look closely at the thigh and deltoid muscle groups for any twitching or fasciculation (look for at least 30 seconds, as these are erratic in their distribution.
d) Tremor- note the character of any tremor. Is it present at rest (Parkinson's) or is movement required to exacerbate it (cerebellar)
e) Scars- of arthrodesis, tendon release, sural nerve biopsy. Don't forget the often overlooked sites of the neck (cervical discectomy), lumbar spine and scalp (aneurysm surgery or ventriculo-peritoneal shunt)
f) Deformity- there may be deformity as result of neurological imbalance, with gross discrepancies in the size of limbs (infantile hemiplegia, childhood polio). The pseudo-hypertrophy seen in both Duchenne and Becker muscular dystrophy is due to replacement of muscle by fatty/fibrous tissue. The classical 'inverted champagne bottle' (greater muscle loss distally than proximally), appearance attributed to Hereditary sensorimotor neuropathy (Charcot-Marie-Tooth) can be seen in any longstanding peripheral neuropathy, as can the often co-existent pes cavus and hammer toe deformities (also Refsum's, Friedrich's ataxia). The deformity of a spastic upper motor neurone syndrome should not be missed (flexed upper limb, extended lower limb), as often this sole finding when unilateral puts the site of the pathology within the cerebral cortex.
g) Mobility- note any surrounding aids to mobility (wheelchair, stick, frame) and the presence of a catheter stand (if the tube itself is not obvious)

2.7.3 Examination Routine for the Neurological System
a) Pronator drift- ask the patient to hold out their arms in front, with the palms facing the ceiling. If the arm starts to drift (often first) and pronate, there is a high chance of detecting other signs of an upper motor neuron (UMN) syndrome.

b) Tone- examine the tone in the arms and legs in the muscle groups either side of the main joints (shoulder, elbows, wrist, hip, knee, ankle). There should be anti-gravity tone present, else hypotonia is evident. If there is increased tone, determine if this can be overcome (spastic) or if this is persistent throughout the movement (extra-cortical).

c) Clonus- it is easiest to perform the test for clonus at this stage for two reasons. Firstly, if present it implies that there is an upper motor neurone problem and hyper-reflexia should be present and secondly it is often forgotten about, if left till later to perform. Clonus is best elicited at either the ankle or knee joint

d) Coordination- again if performed early, valuable information can be sought even before power is assessed. This is particular useful, as occasionally the examiner will cut short your examination if he/she feels that too much time has been taken up by power assessment and an assessment of coordination cannot be made. However, it is extremely unlikely that an examiner will ask you to finish prior to assessing the power. Secondly, if the patient is unable to lift his arm or leg in order to assess coordination, then all that remains to be done when assessing power, is to determine to what degree, the loss of power is. In the upper limb perform the finger-nose test and in the lower limb perform the heel-shin test.

You should be able to differentiate sensory from cerebellar co-ordination by repeating with eyes closed, and noting that coordination is worse with the former (also Romberg's test).

e) Power- assessment of power should be performed with the MRC grading system in mind (0-no movement;1-only a flicker; 2-no anti-gravity power; 3-anti-gravity power but no more; 4-action against gravity; 5-normal power) for all the major flexor/extensor pairs as well as the small muscle of the hand. Once again this should be done in a systematic manner either proximal to distal or vice-versa, and by comparing the muscle groups on each side.

f) Reflexes- with the tendon hammer held perpendicular to the line of the tendon, strike the tendon gently by holding the hammer by its length, in order to ensure a reasonable arc. If you are unable to elicit a reflex, attempt to achieve it with reinforcement (teeth clenching or similar). Remember you are not just looking for the swinging limb, but the contraction of the muscle itself! The reflexes should be graded against the MRC standard (0-areflexia; 1-with reinforcement only; 2-physiological; 3-hyper-reflexic; 4-clonus). Finger jerks may also be demonstrable in hyper-reflexia

g) Inverted supinator jerk- this is loss of the normal brachioradialis contraction that accompanies the finger flexion when the supinator jerk is elicited, and is present when there is a lower motor neuron lesion at C5 and an upper motor neuron lesion below C5 (spondylosis, syrinx, cord tumour)

h) Plantar response- with an orange stick, determine the plantar response. The Babinski response is present if a contraction in the quadriceps is seen, even if the toes don't fan or extend.

i) Hoffman's Reflex- a fairly rare sign in an upper motor neuron (UMN) syndrome; it is performed by grasping the patient's hand with your left hand and with your right index finger stabilising the distal inter-phalangeal joint of the patient's index finger, from below, with your thumb a quick flick of the patient's distal phalanx of the index finger should be performed. Any concomitant flexion of the thumb indicates a positive finding. When present it is a very sensitive sign of an UMN syndrome

j) Sensation- it is important that you are confident about the dermatome distribution in the upper and lower limbs, bearing in mind that the clearest delineation is distally, rather than proximally, and that you are clear in your instructions to the patient. For this reason start distally and assess sensation (start with the orange stick if available, rather than your finger) in the dermatome distribution, working your way proximally. Establish what the patient recognises as normal (i.e reference at the chin), and ask him/her to confirm when they next feel the same again. If you are asked to examine to perform a sensory neurological examination of the lower limbs, the first thing to rule out is a peripheral neuropathy (as this is one of the commonest examine cases). This can be done quickest by assessing vibration loss with the vibrating tuning fork applied to the bony prominence of the metatarsal head, malleoli, patella and if required anterior superior iliac spine. If you cannot detect a peripheral neuropathy then you must resort to performing an orthodox sensory examination as described. Ensure that, if given the time, you perform sufficient tests to determine function in the two main sensory tracts (this usually means 'pin prick' and 'vibration' testing). If during the course of your sensory assessment, there is a gross sensory loss that is bilaterally symmetrical then proceed to determine if a sensory level exists.

k)   Sphincter function- you should enquire about bladder and bowel function by asking the examiner, but along with the obvious catheter tube, sphincter disturbances should be suspected in patients with impaired 'saddle region' anaesthesia

2.7.4 Rapid Assessment List for Neuro Examination:
-   Visual survey- tremor, fasciculations, scars, contractures, wheelchair, stick/cane
-   Assess gait
-   Upper limbs
    -   Check for pronator drift
    -   Check tone
    -   Test coordination (motor & sensory)
    -   Test power in all muscle groups either proximal to distal (or vice-versa)
    -   Reflexes (biceps, triceps, supinator, finger jerks, Hoffman's)
    -   Sensation (distal to proximal)
-   Lower limbs
    -   Check tone
    -   Check for ankle/patella clonus
    -   Test coordination (motor & Sensory)
    -   Test power in all muscles proximal to distal (or vice-versa)
    -   Reflexes (crossed-adductor, knee, ankle & plantar)
    -   Sensation (distal to proximal)
    -   Ask about sphincter function/check anal tone

2.7.5 Common cases in Neurology

2.7.5.1 Peripheral (Sensory) Neuropathy:
-   Look for ulcers, roughened, thickened callous skin
-   Bilateral symmetrical sensory loss to vibration sense (earliest) ± other modalities (later on), starting distally and extending proximally.
-   Motor loss may be present in mixed motor/sensory neuropathies

2.7.5.2 Parkinsonism:
-   Monotonous tone/dysarthria/dysphonia
-   Withdrawn facies
-   ±Supranuclear gaze palsy
-   Asymmetrical resting tremor
-   Bradykinesia
-   Muscle rigidity throughout range of movement (with tremor= cogwheeling)
-   Festinant gait

2.7.5.3 Stroke:
- Asymmetrical facial droop
- Dysphasia
- Circumducting gait
- Spasticity (clasp-knife)
- Hemiparesis
- Asymmetrical hyper-reflexia
- Unilateral extensor plantar response

2.7.5.4 Spastic paraparesis:
- Urinary catheter in situ
- Wheelchair by bedside
- Bilateral symmetrical paralysis of the lower limbs
- Symmetrical lower limb hyper-reflexia
- Bilateral extensor plantar responses
- Sensory level to mid thoracic region

2.7.5.5 Motor neurone disease:
- Dysarthria (pseudobulbar palsy), dysphonia
- Wheelchair/stick
- Fasciculations
- Mixed upper and lower motor neurone signs (spasticity with areflexia or flaccidity with hyper-reflexia)
- No sensory deficits

2.8 Examination of the cranial nerves

2.8.1 Inspection – General
a) Ramsay-Hunt Syndrome- Herpes zoster visible in the outer ear, together with a facial palsy and/or hearing loss
b) Benign Intracranial hypertension- short, obese, hairy women with papilloedema
c) Acromegaly- associated visual field defects
d) Grave's Disease- impaired extra-ocular movements secondary to nerve palsy

2.8.2 Inspection – Specific
a) Ptosis- seen with both Horner's syndrome, and III nerve palsy
b) Shingles-reactivation of latent trigeminal nucleus zoster may be associated with dysaesthesia
c) Props- book with large print, or cane (blind), hearing aid
d) Exophthalmos- when gross will result in impaired ocular movements

2.8.3 Examination Routine for the Cranial Nerves
Examine systematically working through the cranial nerves
a) I & IX (olfactory/glossopharyngeal)- "Has there been a change in the sense of smell or taste?"- suspect anterior cranial fossa floor fracture, frontal tumour, infection or Kallman Syndrome (genetic cause of anosmia and infertility)
b) II (optic)- start by establishing what the level of visual acuity is (Snellen) and then exclude red-green colour blindness (Ishihara), as patients with demyelinating disease may have obvious impairment in both. If visual acuity is impaired; is this correctable with spectacles or a pin hole? If you think the patient is near-blind, then establish if movement and light can be detected. Assess the visual fields by comparing the patient's with your own. Ask the patient to look at your nose, and while you cover one eye determine if the visual field of the other is within the limits of your own. It is best for you to close your ipsilateral eye and for you to cover the patient's ipsilateral eye, to ensure that that eye is completely covered. Next assess the pupillary reflexes; the direct and indirect (consensual) light and near-far accommodation reflexes with a bright pen torch. Determine if there is a relative afferent papillary reflex (greater constriction with a consensual response than a direct light response). Perform fundoscopy by first looking at the anterior chamber then the lens and finally the retina itself. Is there disc cupping (glaucoma) or blurring of the otherwise clear margins (papilloedema)? Are the discs pale (optic atrophy)? Are there any retinal changes of diabetes or hypertension?
c) III, IV & VI (occulomotor, trochlear & abducens)- best assessed together by asking the patient to focus on your finger (kept about a metre away) as it moves to horizontal and vertical extremes noting the full range of movement in each eye, and asking the patient if there is any 'double vision'. If the patient does see double establish which eye's movement is responsible by covering each eye in turn at the point of double vision. The eye from which the most distant image disappears, when covered is the one with the impaired muscle. So on looking right, if when the right eye is covered the most distant image disappears then it is the right lateral rectus that is impaired indicating a dysfunction of the right VIth nerve. Is there nystagmus? If there is, in which plane is it and what is the direction of the fast component? At this time it also best to examine for an inter-nuclear ophthalmoplegia (failure of adduction in one eye and nystagmus in the abducting eye)
d) V (trigeminal) - the ophthalmic and maxillary divisions carry only sensory fibres, the mandibular division carries additional motor fibres. Test for jaw opening, teeth clenching and horizontal jaw translocation, along with sensation in the face (know

the quintothalamic distribution). Inform the examiner that you would like to assess the corneal reflex.

e) VII (facial)- complete ipsilateral facial muscle weakness (above and below brow) indicates a lower motor neuron type lesion. Loss of function confined to below the brow indicates an upper motor neuron type lesion, as above the brow there is a bilateral crossed supra-nuclear input. [Demyelinating disease may result in both types; the latter arising if a large plaque compresses the lower motor nuclear fibre as they emerge from the pons.

f) VIII (vestibular-cochlear) formally requires assessment by performing Weber's and Rinne's tests, but grossly can be determined by the 'Whisper test', whilst occluding the contralateral ear. Note if impairment is associated with VII nerve loss, is highly suggestive of a lesion at the cerebello-pontine angle.

g) IX & X (glossopharyngeal & vagus)- ask to assess the gag reflex

h) XI (accessory)- assess shoulder shrug (trapezius) and movement against resistance of sternocleidomastoid.

i) XII (hypoglossal)- note the size, symmetry, presence of any fasciculations and movement of the tongue. Confirm normal power by asking the patient to push their cheek out with their tongue against your resistance.

2.9 Examination of speech

The physiology of speech consists of three distinct aspects; phonation (generation of noise through the vocal cords), articulation (of the noise into comprehensible sounds) and language and understanding (fluency, comprehension, word formation etc). Therefore, abnormalities in either of these processes (dysphonia, dysarthria & dysphasia) may yield a speech abnormality, and when faced with a case in the exam, though the latter aspect is the most likely to require assessment, you must be able to assess speech in its entirety.

a) Dysphonia- can the patient generate the effort to push air through the vocal cords (myasthenia and other neuromuscular conditions-normal at first but starts to fade), or is there an obstruction within the larynx, or the recurrent laryngeal nerve impeding adequate phonation.

b) Dysarthria- are the words fluent or stuttery? Can the patient pronounce vowels correctly "EE" or "AA" other useful ones are "P" and "B". Are there gross articulation problems when coordination of speech is tested "British constitution" etc (cerebellar). Does the articulation sound mumbling (Parkinson's-also dysphonia)?

c) Dysphasia- this should be assessed in terms of object naming (nominal), fluency & repetition (expressive) and comprehension e.g. by asking the patient to perform simple commands (receptive). Finally, remember that dysphasic speech problems usually imply a lesion in the left (dominant) fronto-temporal region, and other complimentary signs should be sought (right hemiparesis). The presence of a dysphasia will also suggest a cortical lesion when faced with a patient with what looks like a stroke, rather than a lacunar syndrome (internal capsule).

2.10 Examination of fundi

It is helpful to have your own ophthalmoscope with which you are familiar.

Most people find ophthalmoscopy difficult because they become lost and disorientated within the eye. If you take the time to position yourself and the patient correctly and follow the technique outlined below you should find it easier to navigate your way around the fundus and identify pathology in a systematic fashion.

It is important to get an idea of the patients' visual acuity so that you can modify your instructions to the patient if necessary, help you to anticipate what you may see and will also aid you in formulating a final differential diagnosis.
Introduce yourself.

Observe any external signs e.g. nystagmus may be present in a patient with demyelinating disease providing a clue as to the presence of optic atrophy.
Instruct the patient to fix his eyes at a point behind you, which is chosen for height so that you are comfortably able to look into their eye.

Ask for the room to be darkened to facilitate your examination.

Use your right eye to examine the patient's right eye and vice versa. When examining the right eye hold the ophthalmoscope in your right hand and vice versa, placing your index finger on the rotating disc to allow you to alter the power as necessary.

Before looking at the posterior segment start from 50 cm away and look at the red reflex. This provides information about the clarity of the media in front of the retina, such as the presence of cataracts or vitreous haemorrhage, which will be of some diagnostic help if the retina is difficult to visualize.

Move closer to the eye and look at the cornea, anterior chamber, lens and vitreous in turn. Opacities in any of these media will appear as black spots against the red reflex.

The optic disc (blind spot) is located 20 degrees of the visual angle medial/nasal to the macula (center of fixation). It also lies just below the horizontal.

Look into the eye from about 20 degrees lateral/temporal to the line of fixation and from just below the horizontal meridian. The optic disc should come into view immediately and you need to adjust the power of the ophthalmoscope to obtain a sharp image. Check for cupping, colour (pallor/ neovascularisation/ haemorrhages) and contour (swelling/drusen). If the patient's eyes have not been dilated for the examination the abnormality is usually located at the optic disc.

Next follow each of the four major vascular arcades looking for abnormalities such as arterio-venous crossings, vessel caliber and tortuosity.

Examine the peripheral retina in the four quadrants by asking the patient to look in the direction of each quadrant. Look for the presence of pigmentary abnormalities, exudates, haemorrhages and new vessels.

Examine the macula by asking the patient to look at the light of the ophthalmoscope. The macula in health is darker that the surrounding retina in colour and free of blood vessels at its center. It is located one to two disc diameters lateral and a little below the temporal margin of the optic disc. The central depression, the fovea should be identified. Abnormalities in this region will affect visual acuity. Look for exudates, haemorrahges or drusen.

Make sure you don't stop after finding one abnormality, as there may be more. For example hypertensive and diabetic retinopathy frequently coexist and patients with central retinal vein occlusion may have diabetes, hypertension or glaucoma.

The following is a summary of fundal changes in common conditions:

2.10.1 Diabetic Retinopathy

The terminology for diabetic retinopathy is gradually changing following the Early Treatment in diabetic Retinopathy Study, as shown below. However at present for the purposes of the MRCP examination use of the old terminology is acceptable.

Old descriptive term	New term (ETDRS)
Background	Mild non-proliferative diabetic retinopathy (NPDR)
	Moderate NPDR
Pre-proliferative	Severe NPDR
	Very severe NPDR
Proliferative	Proliferative DR
Maculopathy (diffuse, exudative, ischaemic) significant macular oedema)	Maculopathy (Laser treatment based on presence of clinically

Referral times to ophthalmologist, treatment and follow up of different grades of diabetic retinopathy

	Referral time in newly diagnosed patient (wks)	Treatment	Follow-up (months)
Background	13	Nil.	12
Pre-proliferative	6	Nil.	Moderate NPDR: 6-8 Severe NPDR: 3-4
Proliferative	2	Panretinal photocoagulation.	2-3
Maculopathy	6	Focal laser treatment.	2-3

Features:

Clinical classification according to the types of lesions detected on fundoscopy is as follows:

- Mild non-proliferative DR /Background diabetic retinopathy
- Microaneurysms only
- Moderate non-proliferative DR
- More than just microaneurysms but less severe than severe non-proliferative (pre-proliferative) DR. The following may be seen:
- Dot and blot or flame shaped haemorrhages
- Hard exudates
- Cotton-wool spots

Severe non-proliferative DR /Pre-proliferative diabetic retinopathy

Any of the following:
- More than 20 intra-retinal haemorrhages in each of 4 quadrants;
- Venous beading in 2+ quadrants;
- Intraretinal microvascular abnormalities (IRMA) in 1+ quadrant;
- No signs of proliferative DR

Proliferative diabetic retinopathy

One or more of the following:
Neovascularization of the retina, optic disc or iris
Vitreous haemorrhage
Pre retinal haemorrhage
+/- Retinal detachment
+/- Fibrous tissue adherent to vitreous face of retina

Maculopathy

Clinically significant macular oedema (CSME)
Ischaemic Maculopathy (untreatable)
CSME, which appears as retinal thickening, is difficult to appreciate without the aid of binocular vision. Warning signs include hard exudates (circinate if in the form of rings), which indicate oedema and multiple haemorrhages indicating the presence of ischemia.

The **diabetic control and complications trial** was a 6.5-year study into the effects of tight glucose control on microvascular complications in type I diabetic patients. Patients maintained on intensive insulin regime achieved a mean HBA1c of 6.5%. The effect was a 76% reduction in the development of diabetic retinopathy, 54% reduction in the progression of retinopathy, 35-56% reduction in diabetic nephropathy and 60% reduction in diabetic neuropathy.

The **UK Prospective Diabetes Study** was a 10-year study into the effects of tight glucose control on the micro and macro-vascular complications in newly diagnosed type II diabetic patients. Patients maintained on intensive glycaemic control achieved a mean HBA1c of 7.0%. Progression of retinopathy was reduced by 21% and nephropathy by 34%. The UKPDS also found that intensive Blood pressure control (<150/85) reduced the incidence of retinopathy by 35%.

2.10.2 Optic Atrophy

Features:

Degeneration of the nerve fibre bundles of the optic nerve and their replacement by glial cells leads to the pale appearance of the optic disc.

Certain characteristics can give a clue as to the cause. In optic nerve disease (primary optic atrophy) the edges of the disc will be well defined, in contrast to chronic papilloedema where the edge of the disc is indistinct or blurred. In glaucoma the blood vessels will appear to dip at the edge of a cupped optic disc.

To confirm your findings examine for **associated clinical signs**:
- Central scotoma
- Abnormalities of colour perception
- A relative afferent pupillary defect, in unilateral optic neuropathy

Causes:

A. Primary optic atrophy:

1. Demyelination- patient may be young, ask to examine the central visual field and the cerebellar system.
2. Compression by tumour (pituitary, meningioma), aneurysm or Paget's disease. Look for a bitemporal hemianopia and acromegalic facies.
3. Glaucoma (older patient).
4. Ischaemic optic neuropathy, causes for which include central retinal artery occlusion due to thromboembolism (examine the pulse and listen for carotid bruits), giant cell arteritis (palpate the temporal arteries and look for the scar of a temporal artery biopsy) or idiopathic acute anterior ION.
5. Toxins: methanol, tobacco, lead, arsenic, quinine.
6. Nutritional: vitamin B12 deficiency and hyperglycaemia (diabetes)
7. Hereditary: Leber's optic neuropathy (young male), Friedreich's ataxia (look for cerebellar signs, pyramidal lower limb weakness and pes cavus.
8. Trauma including birth hypoxia.
9. Infection: meningitis, encephalitis, and neurosyphilis.

B. Secondary optic atrophy is due to any cause of chronic papilloedema

C. Consecutive optic atrophy is caused by extensive retinal disease such as retinitis pigmentosa and chorioretinitis.

2.10.3 Hypertensive Retinopathy

Features:

Keith-Wagner-Barker classification based on the severity and duration of hypertension:

Grade I	Generalized arteriolar attenuation
Grade II	Severe grade I changes
	Vessel tortuosity
	A-V nipping
	Varying vessel calibre
	Partial concealment of venous blood column
Grade III	Severe grade II changes
	Flame shaped haemorrhages
	Hard exudates +/- Macular star
	Cotton wool spots
Grade IV	Severe grade III changes
	Accelerated/malignant
	Optic disc swelling
	Hypertension

Note that silver and copper wiring as well as arteriovenous crossing changes can be seen in arteriosclerotic retinopathy in the absence of hypertension.

Ask the examiner to check the patient's blood pressure and look for evidence of end-organ damage such as proteinuria and left ventricular hypertrophy.

Mention a few causes of hypertension:

Essential hypertension- 90% of patients

10% of patients have an underlying cause (may be a younger patient):

- Renal
- Endocrine
- Eclampsia
- Coarctation of the aorta

2.10.4 Retinitis Pigmentosa (Rp)

Three main features of this bilateral condition:

1. Retinal pigmentary changes in a bone-spicule pattern.
2. Attenuated retinal vessels
3. Pale optic disc

The pigment conceals the course of retinal vessels. This is in contrast to choroidoretinitis where the vessels can be traced over the areas of hyperpigmentation. There may be atrophic or cystoid Maculopathy.

Also look for associated findings such as optic disc drusen, optic disc cupping and cataracts. Test for peripheral constriction of the visual fields. You should enquire about a history of night blindness and take a family history.

RP is a slow degenerative disorder of the rod photoreceptors with the cones affected late in the disease. It begins in childhood and most patients a registered blind by age 40. Central vision is lost be the seventh decade.

Patterns of inheritance in typical RP:
- Autosomal recessive (51%)
- Autosomal dominant (26%)
- X-linked recessive (23%)

Secondary RP/Systemic associations:
- Phytanic acid storage disease (Refsum's disease)
- Kearns-Sayre syndrome
- Abetalipoprotienaemia (Bassen-Kornweig syndrome)
- Friedreich's ataxia
- Laurance-Moon-Bardet-Biedle syndrome
- Usher's syndrome
- Cockayne's syndrome
- Mucopolysaccharidosis (Hurler's, Hunter's and Sanfilippo's syndromes)

Be prepared to discuss the clinical features of 1 or 2 of these disorders in detail.

Pseudo-RP:
- Trauma
- Posterior ocular inflammation (syphilis, rubella)
- Drug toxicity
- Following central retinal artery occlusion

Management:
- Essential to exclude and treat associated systemic disease.
- For example Refsum's disease is treatable by eliminating phytates (present in dairy products and green vegetables) from the patient's diet.
- Individuals with Refsum disease present with neurologic damage, cerebellar degeneration, and peripheral neuropathy. Onset is most commonly in childhood/adolescence with a progressive course, although periods of stagnation or remission occur. Symptoms also include ataxia, scaly skin (ichthyosis), difficulty hearing, and eye problems including cataracts and night blindness.
- An ECG can be like saving in a patient's with Kearn-Sayre syndrome, as it will detect heart block requiring pacemaker insertion.
- Genetic counselling.
- Blind registration and low visual aid assessment.

2.10.5   Papilloedema

This is a specific term relating to swollen discs secondary to **raised intracranial pressure**.

Features:
- Bilateral
- Disc hyperaemia
- Indistinct margins
- Absence of spontaneous venous pulsation
- Dilated veins
- Splinter haemorrhages, cotton wool spots and hard exudates
- Optic atrophy (late stage)

Papilloedema does not always occur with raised intracranial pressure (ICP). When present ICP has been raised for at least 24 hours. Visual acuity is usually good with normal colour vision but there may be enlargement of the blind spot. Following normalization of ICP papilloedema takes up to 8 weeks to resolve.

Contrast this with papillitis:
- Maybe unilateral
- Reduced visual acuity
- Reduced colour vision
- Presence of an RAPD
- Signs of associated systemic disease e.g. demyelination, TB, sarcoid
- Evidence of intraocular inflammation (vitreous cells)

Causes of Papilloedema:
- Intracranial space occupying lesion (tumour, abscess, haematoma)
- Malignant hypertension
- Idiopathic intracranial hypertension
- Meningitis
- Cerebral anoxia
- Aqueduct stenosis or other cause of hydrocephalus
- Sagittal sinus thrombosis

Causes of optic disc swelling:
- Papilloedema
- Optic neuritis/papillitis
- Ischaemic optic neuropathy
- Malignant hypertension
- Central retinal vein occlusion
- Toxic, hereditary, compressive optic neuropathy
- Diabetic papillitis
- Pseudo-swelling of infiltrative optic neuropathy

2.10.6   Old Choroidoretinitis

Features:
Scars of old choroidoretinitis appear as well-defined white patches (where the retina is atrophic) with pigmented edges (due to proliferation of the retinal pigment epithelium). The blood vessels can be seen to pass over the lesions undisturbed.

Differential diagnosis of pigmented retina:
- Normal racial variant
- Malignant melanoma
- Retinitis pigmentosa
- Scars of pan-retinal photocoagulation

Causes of Choroidoretinitis:
- Cytomegalovirus
- Congenital toxoplasmosis
- Toxocara
- AIDS

- Sarcoidosis
- Behcet's disease
- TB
- Syphilis

2.10.7   Retinal Vein Thrombosis

Features of branch retinal vein occlusion:
- Tortuosity of occluded vein, most commonly the supratemporal vein.
- Dot and blot haemorrhages and cotton wool spots surrounding the occluded vein.
- The obstruction occurs distal to the arteriovenous crossing
- +/- macular oedema

Look for evidence of hypertensive or diabetic retinopathy and glaucomatous optic disc changes.

Features of central retinal vein occlusion:
- Generalized retinal vein engorement and tortuosity.
- Dot and blot and flame shaped haemorrhages in all four quadrants.
- Multiple cotton wool spots.
- Optic disc swelling in the acute stage.
- Disc collateral vessels, retinal exudates, arterial and venous sheathing in the chronic stages.

Risk factors:
- Hypertension
- Raised intraocular pressure
- Diabetes
- Hyperviscosity syndromes
- Retinal periphlebitis e.g. sarcoidosis, behcet's disease
- Collagen vascular diseases

Management:
Investigate and treat underlying systemic disease (fellow eye is at risk).

Refer to an ophthalmologist within 2-3 weeks. Principles of management lie in prevention of neovascularisation (rubeotic glaucoma typically occurs within 3 months of occlusion) and macular oedema.

Fluorescein angiography will define the degree of ischemia and hence risk of neovascularisation. Retinal ischemia or macular oedemas are treated by laser photocoagulation.

Patients are seen regularly to check for signs of ischemia (cotton-wool spots, iris and disc new vessels).

2.10.8   Myelinated Optic Disc

A benign congenital abnormality known as medullated or myelinated nerve fibres. Myelination begins in fetal life at the lateral geniculate body reaching the optic disc at birth. In 1% of the population myelination does not stop at the lamina cribrosa but extends onto the nerve fibres surrounding the optic disc.

Features:
The optic disc contains a white irregular streaky patch. The myelination may extend from the disc and terminate peripherally in a feather-like pattern. It usually obscures the retinal vessels.

Look for other clinical findings associated with myelinated optic disc:
- Enlargement of the blind spot
- Variable visual field loss depending on the extent of myelination
- Amblyopia (reduced visual acuity in affected eye)
- Myopia

2.10.9　　Retinal Artery Occlusion

Features of central retinal artery occlusion:
- Reduced visual acuity
- An RAPD
- The retinal artery shows cattle-tracking (stagnation of the circulation with clumping of the blood within the arteriole)
- Cotton wool spots
- Cherry red spot at the fovea. This is the intact choroidal circulation which is visible where the retina is at its thinnest and stands out against the ischaemic milky white macula. It disappears after 2 weeks.
- In chronic cases there is retinal atrophy, arteriolar narrowing and optic atrophy.

N.B a few differential diagnoses for a cherry red spot at the macula:
- The sphingolipidoses. Deposition of GM2 gangliosidase with the retinal ganglion cells gives the retina its pale colour and as these calls are sparse at the fovea, the red colour of the underlying choroidal circulation is seen in sharp contrast to the surrounding retina.
- Quinine toxicity
- Traumatic retinal oedema

Features of branch artery occlusion:
- Sectoral visual field defect
- Sectoral retinal ischaemia and changes as above
- An embolus may be visible

Causes of retinal artery occlusion:
- Emboli from the heart or stenosed carotids arteries.
  - There are three main varieties of **emboli**:
    - Cholesterol (Hollenhorst plaque) arising from the carotid arteries.
    - Platelet-fibrin emboli associated with large vessel arteriosclerosis.
    - Calcific emboli arising from cardiac valves.
- Vaso-obliterative disorders e.g. atherosclerosis or vasculitides (giant cell arteritis, collagen vascular diseases).
- Excessively high intraocular pressure (angle closure glaucoma, post retinal detachment surgery)

Management:
This is an ophthalmic emergency. An ophthalmologist must see the patient within 48 hours of the onset of symptoms, as treatment with in this time can improve visual outcome.
Remember that retinal artery occlusions are similar to cerebral CVAs or TIAs and thus treatment and investigations are very similar:

Tell the examiner you wish to check the patient's blood pressure and perform a cardiovascular examination in order to exclude an irregular pulse, a carotid bruit and a heart murmur.

Investigations and Management
- Initiate anti-platelet therapy
- Request an ESR +/- temporal artery biopsy
- Treatment of co-existing hypertension, diabetes and hyperlipidaemia
- Perform Carotid doppler ultrasound, ECG, echocardiogram.

2.10.10   Age-Related Maculopathy And Macular Degeneration

Features:
- Bilateral disease unusually affecting patients over the age of 65.
- Two types dry or non-exudative and wet or exudative.
- Multiple drusen (colloid bodies) at the macula. These are yellow-white and slightly elevated. The retinal vessels can be seen to travel over them compared with hard exudates, which obscure the vessels.
- Hard drusen are small, round and discrete. These are usually innocuous and seen in age related maculopathy.
- Soft drusen are larger and have ill-defined edges. They are associated with ARMD.
- Macular pigmentation and hypopigmentation representing atrophy of the retinal pigment epithelium (RPE) (dry type).
- Confluent macular pigmentation known as geographic atrophy.
- Subretinal haemorrhages (due to choroidal neovascularisation) +/- macular elevation due to RPE detachment (wet type).
- Disciform scar at the macula. Well-defined white-yellow palque.
- There is loss central vision with intact peripheral visual field.

ARMD is the commonest cause of blind registration in the UK today. Certain types of wet ARMD based on angiographic criteria are amiable to laser treatment.

2.10.11   Angioid Streaks

Features:
- Dark brown streaks with serrated edges, radiating out from the optic disc.
- Deep to the retinal vessels.
- Darker and wider that retinal vessels.

Streaks are due to cracks in Bruch's membrane.

Systemic associations are found in 50% of patients:
- Pseudoxanthoma elasticum
- Paget's disease
- Sickle cell anaemia
- Ehlers-Danlos syndrome
- Thrombocytopenic purpura
- Marfan's syndrome
- Acromegaly
- Lead poisoning

2.11 PACES Exam Tips

1. Appearance- come to the exam dressed smartly and appropriately, with well-groomed hair, tied back if likely to fall in front of you whilst examining patients.

2. Composure- maintain your cool despite how intimidating the examiners appear. Do not engage in fruitless discussions with the examiners about whether certain signs are present or absent. This is entirely pointless and wastes your time and increases the examiner's irritability. You may of course be right, but going down this path is likely to fluster you for the remainder of the examination.

3. Politeness- always greet the patient with a hello and introduction, seeking their permission to examine them, and complete your examination by thanking them. This is also not a bad idea when dealing with the examiners.

4. Methodology- be thoughtful in how you are going to approach examining the patient in front of you, in light of what your instructions are. Always start by establishing that the patient does not have any pain in the region of interest, and if they do be gentle in your examination. Keep looking at the patient whilst you palpate/percuss to see if you are hurting them; you should know where your hands are without having to look at them and the last thing you need is the patient quietly grimacing to the examiner whilst you examine them. There is no point in performing an orthodox comprehensive examination if both your written instruction and your examiner ask you to concentrate on one particular aspect. You are not going to get any additional credit for doing this. Whilst examining think about the signs you have so far detected and try and put them together in your mind as you complete the rest of the examination.

    Often this will make interpretation at the end easier and will also give you an idea of what the expected finding is, even before performing the specific test. For example if you have elicited ankle clonus when assessing tone in the lower limb, when you come to test the reflexes, you will be expecting to find hyper-reflexia.

5. Presentation- when you have finished examining the patient, turn to the examiner, and don't look back at the patient. Stand straight with arms by your side or in front and not in your pockets!

    Be confident. Be clear and fluent in what you say, as hesitancy doesn't inspire confidence; and be prepared to justify any diagnosis that you offer. Either offer a diagnosis (especially if that is what you were asked to do) and support it with your findings, or if a diagnosis or diagnoses are not clearly obvious to you, present your findings. Your examiner is likely to let you know early on which he/she requires.

    If there were unexpected findings which have made you refute a diagnosis that you were considering then it is reasonable to offer the diagnosis to the examiner, explaining which of your findings were seemingly at odds with it. Although, your suggested diagnosis may be incorrect, at least you will have made some logical interpretation of your findings. Conversely, it is foolish to offer a diagnosis which is at complete odds with your findings and, one which you could not justify if asked to do so.

Lastly, don't attempt to cover up omissions or make up signs! Although it may seem at this stage that you have omitted a major part of the examination, it is better to admit to doing so. Remember the examiner has been there with you whilst you examined the patient, and he/she will have noted your omission.

6.   Discussion- after you have presented your findings, and if there is time, you may be asked a few questions regarding the case at hand. These may include other possible differential diagnoses, or investigations that could be performed to confirm your diagnosis. Additionally, you may be asked how you would manage the care of the patient. When answering these questions, be concise and don't recite paragraphs from textbooks, in an attempt to disguise an inability to answer the question.

7.   Be graceful-there are no extra points in arguing with the examiner about how he/she is wrong because you read a more modern review on the train journey that morning. You may be right, but if you are at a stage where those sorts of issues are arising in your examination, then it is likely that you are doing well. There is no need to go overboard, and annoy the examiner.

3 HISTORY TAKING SKILLS

What is expected from the candidate?
- The history taking skills station aims to assess the candidate's ability to gather relevant facts from the patient, assimilate this information and then discuss the case with, appropriate clinical guidance for the patient.
- In the Paces exam, the candidate will be given written instructions for the case, usually in the form of either a GP or specialist nurse letter, or a clinic letter from a previous recent hospital outpatient's clinic.
- The clinical situation could be an out patients appointment, or a history taken in casualty.
- The candidate will be given this information during a five-minute interval before the start of the station.
- 15 minutes are allowed for the history taking followed by 5 minutes for discussion; The patient will be asked to leave the station prior to this.
- The 2 examiners are present throughout observing the history taking. Ideally they will have been asked to sit behind you or out of view. Each examiner has a structured mark sheet for the case.
- You will be marked on your history taking technique as well as your ability to establish key relevant facts from the patient regarding the problem at hand. You will also need to establish risk factors where necessary and be able to communicate this to the examiners.

Advice to the candidate:
- This is a situation with which you should be entirely familiar after all you will be taking histories in outpatients, A&E, and at the patient bedside many times a day. Approach this station with confidence and use your abilities as a practising doctor to keep yourself and the patient at ease.
- Stay calm and relaxed, the patient has been advised to be helpful so there is no need to worry about detective mysteries.
- Speak clearly and ask direct questions, if you do not understand the patients answer, ask them to elaborate as you would do in a normal clinical setting.
- Remember that you as an SHO are one of the first people to deal with new patients and you will be performing this task more frequently on a day to day basis than your examiners.
- Do not be intimidated by the examiners watching you. Carry on conducting the history taking as if they were not there. Do not keep turning to them for reassurance. This is an opportunity to gain easy marks by demonstrating that you are a confident and competent doctor.
- Remember to follow the history taking protocol and not just jump in to a dead end pathway. After establishing the presenting compliant, go on to establish the history of presenting complaint, the past medical history, drugs, family history, just as you would in clinical practice. There may be points not mentioned in the referral letter that the examiner is expecting you to establish. Drug side effects are commonly used.
- Finish by asking the patient if there are any questions that the patient would wish to ask you.

DO NOT
At any time request or attempt to examine the patient (your examination skills will be assessed in different parts of the examination). Don't even mention examination at this station.

3.1 Case 1

3.1.1 Candidate information

2nd February 2002

Dear Doctor,

Thank you for seeing this 32 year old lady who has been suffering from hot sweats and irritability for three months. She has also lost over a stone in weight.
She has a history of heart disease in her family and her mother had an under active thyroid.

With best wishes

Dr Banks

Instructions to the candidate

You have 14 minutes with the patient and 1 minute for reflection before discussion with the examiners.

Take as detailed a general medical history as possible with emphasis on the cause for complaint

You are not expected to examine the patient.

Case 1

3.1.2 Subject Information:

You are a 28-year-old schoolteacher working in a busy inner city school.

Since returning from the summer holidays, you have found work very stress full and in many instances have been reduced to tears by the actions of demanding students. Your school has also had an OFSTED inspection and you have been working most evenings to ensure that all performance targets are met.

You have felt very hot and have suffered from bouts of diarrhoea and insomnia since the summer.

When you first saw your GP, your symptoms were thought to be caused by anxiety and you were prescribed a small dose of diazepam as a temporary measure to take at night.

In the last three months, you have lost 2 stones in weight, the diarrhoea continues and you feel tearful most of the time. You are exhausted all the time. You finally decided to see the GP again when you had a bout of palpitations whilst crossing the road.

On this occasion you were seen by a different GP who suggested checking your thyroid

Your past medical history consists of migraines for which you have had a brain scan which was normal.

You take a sleeping tablet at night and brufen for headaches.

Your mother had an under active thyroid and had heart problems because of this and you are now also worried that it may affect your heart.

You are allergic to peanuts (your face and lips swell if brought into contact)

You smoke 20 cigarettes a day and drink 3 glasses of red wine at night.

You live with your husband and 2 young children.

Case 1

3.1.3 Examiner information

Problem: Patient who presents with symptoms of thyrotoxicosis

Your observation

1. The candidate will not have access to blood test results confirming thyrotoxicosis.

2. The history should focus on current symptoms with a thorough general review of systems to covey that the candidate is aware of the diverse differential diagnosis for weight loss. They will need to ascertain from the patient that she has lost weight despite having a good appetite and eating vast amounts.

3. The candidate will also need to demonstrate knowledge that they are aware of both the diverse manner that this condition may present itself and also the involvement of the cardiovascular, ocular, gastrointestinal, loco-motor and reproductive systems.

4. There is a family history and Graves' disease is the most likely pathology. Questions should also focus on the search for possible other autoimmune disease such as type 1 diabetes and pernicious anaemia.

5. This lady is a smoker and may be at greater risk of eye disease and the candidate must ask if there has been noticeable bulging of the eyes or double vision.

6. A good candidate will find this case fairly straightforward and will have little problem in establishing a good and thorough history in the time allocated. They should then present the case as a summary at the end.

3.1.4 Tutorial: Thyrotoxicosis

The clinical manifestations of thyrotoxicosis are largely independent of its cause and arise from elevated levels of free thyroid hormones in the blood stream. However, the disorder that is causing the thyrotoxicosis may have additional effects e.g. Graves' disease which as well as causing thyrotoxicosis also has unique problems which are not related to high serum free thyroid hormone concentrations. These problems include ophthalmopathy, pretibial myxoedema and clubbing.

Clinical manifestations of Thyrotoxicosis:

Skin: Warm and sweaty due to vasodilation. There may be associated pruritis, vitiligo, alopecia, onycholysis and pretibial myxoedema.

Gastro-intestinal : Weight loss due to increased calorie burn up due to increased basal metabolic rate, increased gut motility with associated diarrhoea and malabsorption. Most patients have hyperphagia. Anorexia may occur particularly in the elderly. Patients with large goitres may also experience dysphagia.

Cardiovascular: Tachycardia; The cardiac output is increased due to increased peripheral oxygen utilisation and also increased cardiac contractility. High or normal output cardiac failure may occur in severe thyrotoxicosis and pre-existing heart failure may deteriorate.

Atrial fibrillation occurs in 10-20% and is more common in the elderly. In 60% of these the rhythm will spontaneously revert to sinus when the thyrotoxicosis is treated. Mitral valve prolapse is 2-3 times more common in hyperthyroid patients.

Respiratory: Dyspnoea due to increased oxygen consumption, respiratory muscle weakness and tracheal obstruction. Thyrotoxicosis may exacerbate underlying asthma.

Eyes: Only in Graves' disease. There is inflammation of the extra-ocular muscles, orbital fat and connective tissue which result in proptosis and exophthalmos, impairment of eye muscle function and periorbital oedema.

Ophthalmopathy is more common in cigarette smokers.

Patients may complain of a gritty discomfort in the eyes and or diplopia. Corneal ulceration may occur and in severe proptosis, optic neuropathy may lead to blindness.

Skeletal: Thyroid acropachy (clubbing with periosteal new bone formation seen in Graves, osteoporosis in chronic hyperthyroidism.

Neuromuscular: emotional liability, insomnia, irritability, anxiety; Proximal muscle weakness, tremor.

3.2 Case 2

3.2.1 Candidate information

February 2nd 2002

Dear Doctor,

Thank you for seeing this sensitive young man who has recently moved to this area. He is now in his mid-twenties. He suffered a traumatic head injury at the age of seven, which has left him with several problems.

He has confirmed hypogonadism and is troubled by erectile dysfunction.

He has a number of issues, which I am at a loss to answer.

Thank you for assessment

Dr A Barreto

Instructions to the candidate
You have 14 minutes with the patient and 1 minute for reflection before discussion with the examiners.

Take as detailed a general medical history as possible with emphasis on the cause for complaint

You are not expected to examine the patient.

Case 2

3.2.2 Subject Information

Hypogonadism and Erectile dysfunction
You are a 28 year old man.

Your main problems are that you are having great difficulty in maintaining long term relationships with your girlfriends. You feel that this is largely due to some very personal problems that you have had great difficulty in discussing with anyone.

You are unable to have erections despite having been in situations where you have been appropriately aroused mentally. You then make up excuses as to why you cannot sleep with your lovers causing them upset and damaging your relationships.

You were run over at the age of 7 and were in hospital for almost a year with many fractures, leg injuries and severe head injuries. You were told that you would need hormones to help you with puberty and were followed up by some doctors in the children's clinic.

You only developed scanty pubic hair at the age of 17 with the help of some treatment which you think was testosterone by the paediatric doctors at the local hospital in your hometown. They had also given you hormones to help you grow taller. You were getting erections at that time even on waking but you were not sexually active.

At present, you get very weak erections most mornings on waking but not otherwise. You have never noticed any breast milk production but your libido is now low and you feel this may be due to loss of confidence.

You feel tired and sleep all the time and are currently unemployed.

You smoke 12 cigarettes a day and drink about 8 pints a week. You have taken class B drugs from time to time.

You have always been a bit constipated.

You are also becoming more and more depressed and isolated because whilst you initially had the confidence to make friends and girlfriends, you just feel as though it's no use because it never amounts to much.

You are not currently taking any medication although your GP has suggested that you may be offered Testosterone or Viagra by the hospital.

You are quite inpatient and will often interrupt the doctor to get your point across.

Case 2

3.2.3 Examiner information

This is a difficult case due to the combination of

1. A complicated endocrine history

2. A patient who is not entirely able to give the candidate information of the exact treatment that they have had in the past.

In this case you are observing that the candidate

1. Takes a clear history from the patient

2. Is not visibly anxious and uncertain about what to ask to gather facts for a basic medical history. Is able to keep the patient calm and reassured whilst talking about erectile dysfunction.

3. Is able to look for other features of panhypopituitarism such as :
   - Hyperprolactinaemia: Galactorrhoea, reduced libido, headaches
   - Growth Hormone deficiency: Lethargy, weight gain, depression reduced muscle mass, sleepiness
   - Hypothyroidism

4. Remains professional despite numerous interruptions from the patient

5. Is able to take control of the clinical situation

6. Is not fazed by some outrageous questions and answers them professionally.

3.2.4 Tutorial: Hypogonadism

Hypogonadism in a man refers to a reduction in either of the 2 major functions of the testes:
- Sperm production
- Testosterone production

These disorders may result from disease of the testes (Primary Hypogonadism) or disease from the pituitary or hypothalamus (Secondary hypogonadism). In some cases the disorder may result from testosterone insensitivity arising from abnormalities at the testosterone receptor.

The distinction between primary and secondary hypogonadism is made by measurement of serum FSH and LH.

Primary Hypogonadism	Secondary Hypogonadism
Serum Testosterone is low.	Serum Testosterone is subnormal.
Sperm count is low. It is proportionately much lower than the testosterone.	Sperm count is subnormal. It is proportional to the reduction in testosterone.
FSH and LH concentrations are increased and may be very high.	FSH and LH concentrations are normal or reduced.
More likely to be associated with gynecomastia due to effects of FSH & LH on testosterone aromatase which results in increase conversion of testosterone to estradiol.	Gynecomastia does occur but often to a lesser extent.
Causes: Congenital Klinefeltors (XXY), 46 XY/XO , Mutations to the FSH receptor gene, Cryptorchidism, Varicocele, Disorders of Androgen biosynthesis, Myotonic dystrophy	Covered below
Causes: Acquired Infections (mumps), radiation, alkylating and antineoplastic agents, suramin, ketoconazole, trauma, torsion, autoimmune, cirrhosis, chronic renal failure, HIV.	Covered below

Causes of Secondary Hypogonadism in males:

Congenital:

Congenital abnormalities associated with a reduction in gonadotropin secretion are rare but well recognized and easy to diagnose.

- Sexual differentiation in all of these disorders is normal male, because testosterone secretion occurs by the fetal Leydig cells following hCG stimulation cells in the first trimester of pregnancy, when sexual differentiation occurs.

- In contrast, phallic development during the third trimester is subnormal, because testicular testosterone secretion at this stage is dependent upon fetal LH secretion, which is subnormal. This leads to diminished testosterone secretion by the fetal testes, resulting in a small phallus, called micropenis.

- Childhood growth is normal if gonadotropin deficiency is an isolated event, or subnormal if it is associated with impaired growth hormone or thyroid hormone release.

- Pubertal development is diminished or even absent, depending upon the degree of gonadotropin deficiency. Gonadotropin deficiency can occur in the absence of any other abnormalities or can be associated with other hormonal or non-hormonal abnormalities.

1. Isolated idiopathic hypogonadotropic hypogonadism:: This is a Congenital secondary hypogonadism that occurs in the absence of any other abnormalities. It is usually the consequence of GnRH (gonadotropin-releasing hormone) deficiency, as demonstrated by a normal response of serum LH to synthetic GnRH after repetitive administration of synthetic GnRH [However, families have been described who have isolated gonadotropin deficiency as a consequence of mutations of the GnRH receptor.

2. Kallmann's syndrome: Kallmann's syndrome is characterized by hypogonadotropic hypogonadism and one or more non-gonadal congenital abnormalities, including anosmia, red-green color blindness, midline facial abnormalities such as cleft palate, urogenital tract abnormalities and neurosensory hearing loss. Hypogonadism in this syndrome is a result of deficient hypothalamic secretion of GnRH. The hypogonadism may be severe, mild, or even transient. Most cases of Kallmann's syndrome are sporadic, but familial occurrence also occurs. Inheritance is usually X-linked, as judged by the much greater number of cases in males than females. However, autosomal dominant or recessive transmission can occur.

3. Idiopathic hypogonadotropic hypogonadism associated with mental retardation : Several syndromes, such as Prader-Willi syndrome, have been described in which hypogonadotropic hypogonadism is associated with retardation and other abnormalities, including obesity.

4. Abnormal ß-subunit of LH: A rare but instructive cause of hypogonadotropic hypogonadism is caused by a point mutation in the LH ß-subunit gene .This single base pair mutation leads to a single amino acid substitution in the ß-subunit, which in turn results in greatly impaired binding of LH to its receptor on

Leydig cells. The LH therefore has subnormal bioactivity but normal immunoreactivity.

5. Abnormal ß-subunit of FSH: Another rare cause is a mutation in the gene for the ß-subunit of FSH. A man with this mutation had delayed puberty with low serum testosterone and FSH concentrations, but with a high serum LH concentration. The low serum testosterone concentration is hard to explain because the Leydig cells do not have FSH receptors.

Acquired Diseases:

In general, a mass lesion in the pituitary or hypothalamus is more likely to diminish the secretion of gonadotropins than that of ACTH and TSH. Thus, patients may present with hypogonadism without either adrenal or thyroid deficiency.

- Benign tumors and cysts: Any kind of pituitary adenoma or cyst can cause sufficient pressure on the gonadotroph cells to interfere with their function and decrease LH and FSH secretion. In addition, hyperprolactinemia caused by lactotroph adenomas inhibits gonadotropin.

- Malignant tumours: Malignant tumors are more likely to affect the hypothalamus than the pituitary. These include both primary (e.g., meningiomas) and metastatic tumors (e.g., breast in women and lung and prostate in men).

- Infiltrative diseases: Sarcoidosis and Langerhans cell histiocytosis (eosinophilic granuloma) can cause hypothalamic hypogonadism, while iron deposition hemochromatosis can cause pituitary hypogonadism. Treatment of the underlying disease may improve gonadotropin secretion. The age of the patient is important in hemochromatosis, since reversal of hypogonadism with venesection therapy is more likely to occur in men under the age of 40.

- Infections: Meningitis is a rare cause of hypogonadism. Tuberculous meningitis can lead to hypopituitarism.

- Pituitary apoplexy: Sudden and severe haemorrhage into the pituitary can result in permanent impairment of pituitary function, including hypogonadism.

- Trauma : Trauma to the base of the skull can sever the hypothalamic-pituitary stalk and interrupt the portal circulation, thereby preventing GnRH from reaching the gonadotroph cells in the pituitary and decreasing LH and FSH release.

- Critical illness: Any critical illness, such as surgery, myocardial infarction, or head trauma can cause hypogonadotropic hypogonadism.

- Chronic, systemic illness : Several chronic, systemic illnesses, including cirrhosis, chronic renal failure, and AIDS, cause hypogonadism by a combination of primary and secondary effects.

- Glucocorticoid treatment: Chronic treatment with glucocorticoids can lead to hypogonadism.

- Chronic narcotic administration: Chronic narcotic cause pronounced hypogonadism.

- Idiopathic

3.3 Case 3

3.3.1 Candidate information

Dear Doctor,

Thank you for seeing this 34 year old women who has suffered from an eating disorder since her teens.

She came to see my colleague last week complaining of dizziness and fatigue. Her full blood count has shown her to have an Hb of 4.9 with microcytosis.

Please advise

Yours faithfully
Dr Patel

Instructions to the candidate

You have 14 minutes with the patient and 1 minute for reflection before discussion with the examiners.

Take as detailed a general medical history as possible with emphasis on the cause for complaint

You are not expected to examine the patient.

Case 3

3.3.2 Subject information

You are a 34-year-old women who presented on this occasion with gradual onset of severe fatigue over the last 6 months and dizziness independent of posture for 3 weeks, which came on after a heavy period.

You have never felt completely well since your teens.

You were first seen in the paediatric clinic for a condition called PICA when you found yourself eating wall plastering because you got a strange craving for it. You mother was particularly concerned and you were seen by the psychiatrists as well. You were at that time found to be anaemic and this was attributed to your diet and your periods. You were given a diet sheet but you felt like a freak and did not attend hospital appointments after you started university.

You have been working in Australia for 10 years and returned to the UK a year ago.

You have noticed pains in your legs which are in your thighs and you feel as though your bones ache. You have also developed painful ulcers in your mouth. You can't seem to put weight on.

Your stools are a pale yellow and you can't always flush them. They feel greasy and look different to the motions passed by your partner.

You have never had diarrhoea or contact with tropical illness.

You are currently on iron tablets but this has made little difference to your well-being.

There is no illness in your family that you are aware of.

Case 3

3.3.3 Examiner information:

Adult female with coeliac's disease

This lady has presented with symptoms of anaemia.

Her past medical history consists of Pica, which can be a manifestation of anaemia.

She was not formerly investigated for this in her teens partly due to her non-compliance with clinics and partly due to the involvement of the eating disorders team in liaison psychiatry.

She has other features of malabsorption, particularly steatorrhoea, symptomatic vitamin D deficiency (manifested by her return to a cooler climate) and oral ulceration.

1. The candidate must demonstrate a clear understanding of the symptoms of anaemia and ask questions that will furnish all necessary information including a menstrual history.

2. A differential diagnosis must be sort for and coeliac disease should be high on the list.

3.3.4 Tutorial: Coeliac Disease

PICA:
This is a condition characterised by an abnormal appetite for non-food substances such as clay, wood or paper.

PAGOPHAGIA:
This condition is PICA for ice and is considered quite specific for an iron deficiency state. It may present in patients who are not anaemic and responds rapidly with treatment of iron often before any increase is seen in the haemoglobin concentration.

ANAEMIA:
Anaemia is defined as a low haemoglobin due to a reduction in the red cell mass.
Manifestations: The manifestations of iron deficiency occur in several stages.
*   Stage 1:Depletion of iron stores;
*   Stage 2: Development of anaemia with a reduction in the red cell mass initially normocytic
*   Stage 3: Profound anaemia with hypochromia and microcytosis reflective of iron deficient haemopoesis.

Symptoms: Commonly weakness, headaches, tinnitus, irritability and varying degrees of fatigue and exercise intolerance. Many patients are asymptomatic.
Some patients may experience dizziness, palpitations, chest pain shortness of breath, anorexia and bowel disturbance.

Signs: Pallor, hyperdynamic circulation, hypotension, cardiac failure an retinal haemorrhages.

Causes:
- Physiological: Pregnancy
- Blood loss: Menorrhagia, occult bleeding, inflammatory bowel disease, peptic ulcer disease
- Reduced iron absorption: Coeliac disease
- Chronic renal failure, bone marrow failure, hypothyroidism
- Intravascular haemolysis with its accompanying haemoglobinuria and haemosiderinuria can lead to significant losses in patients with paroxysmal nocturnal haemoglobinura
- B12 and folate deficiency

Coeliac Disease: (Gluten sensitive enteropathy)
In this condition, there is a permanent intolerance of gluten which is a wheat protein resulting in gastrointestinal malabsorption and villous atrophy. Although classically a disease of infants, it often presents later between the ages of 10 and 40. When unrecognised, it is associated with a high mortality due to an 8 fold increase in upper GI malignancies and a 20 to 30 fold increase in the risk of intestinal lymphoma. Most deaths are due to Non Hogkins lymphoma.

The classic definition includes the following features:
- Symptoms of malabsorption such as staetorrhea, weight loss or other signs of nutrient or vitamin deficiency
- Villous atrophy
- Resolution of the mucosal lesions and symptoms upon withdrawing gluten containing foods from the diet. This may take up to several months.

The severity of the coeliac intestinal lesion does not necessarily correlate with the severity of the clinical symptoms although there is a gradient of decreasing severity from the proximal to distal small intestine.
Failure to improve on a gluten free diet may be due to poor compliance or other underlying malabsorptive disorders.

The frequent occurrence in first degree relatives and remarkable close association with HLA-DQ2 and or DQ8 gene locus provide the basis of our current understanding that the disease is an immune disorder that is triggered by the gliadin component of gluten in genetically predisposed individuals.

In current practice, serological studies are used to aid diagnosis. These include:
- IgA Endomysial antibody (IgA EMA) which has the highest diagnostic accuracy. It is moderately sensitive and highly specific for coeliacs disease.
- IgA tissue transglutaminase antibody (IgA tTG) which are quite sensitive and specific.
- IgA antigliadin (IgA AGA), gliadin is a component of gluten.

All of these antibody levels fall with effective treatment and as a result they can be used as a non-invasive means of monitoring response to a gluten free diet.

Non GI manifestations of coeliacs:
- Iron deficiency anaemia (12%)
- Arthritis
- Ataxia, epilepsy
- Anxiety, depression
- Metabolic bone

Associated conditions:
- Dermatitis Herpetiformis (85% of patients have coeliacs)
- Type 1 diabetes (7%) due to shared genetic loci HLA – DR3, HLA – DQ2 and the IDDM 3 locus on chromosome 15q26.
- Selective IgA deficiency (8% have coeliacs)
- Downs syndrome (16%)
- Liver disease (non-specific mild elevation of aminotransferase levels although severe liver disease has been documented).
- Autoimmune thyroid disease (hypothyroidism is more frequent).
- Myocarditis and cardiomyopathy although rare has been shown to respond to gluten free diets and immunosuppression.

3.4 Case 4

3.4.1 Candidate information

Dear Doctor,

Thank-you for seeing this 38 year- old woman, with type 2 diabetes. Her control is poor and her most recent HbA1c is 12%.

She complains of blurry vision and pains in her thighs.

Her current treatment regimen is Metformin 500mg bd.

Incidentally her cholesterol is raised at 7.1

Please could you advise.

Dr Kumar

Instructions to the candidate
You have 14 minutes with the patient and 1 minute for reflection before discussion with the examiners.

Take as detailed a general medical history as possible with emphasis on the cause for complaint

You are not expected to examine the patient.

Case 4

3.4.2 Subject Information

You are a 38 year old woman who was diagnosed with type 2 diabetes 5 years ago.

You have had 2 pregnancies at the age of 28 and 31 and were told that your sugar was high at the time but you were able to control it with diet alone.

Your babies were large, both weighing over 10lbs.

You have not been a good attendee to clinics but have become concerned because your thighs ache and your vision has become blurry over the last 6 weeks.

You have not had your eyes checked for several years and you can't sleep due to burning pains in your feet.

You take metformin 500mg bd and a vitamin tablet daily.

Both your parents are diabetic.

You smoke 10 cigarettes a day and drink half a bottle of wine each night.

You work as a chef and you diet and meal times are erratic.

Case 4

3.4.3 Examiner Information

Points to establish in history:
- Duration of type 2 diabetes
- Symptoms on presentation
- When symptoms above began
- Last eye check
- Any notable change in visual acuity
- Specific questions regarding thigh pain (? Amyotrophy)
- Any other symptoms of hyperglycaemia
- Any problems with pain or numbness in the feet
- Current home monitoring
- Any hospital admissions related to diabetes

Candidate should also ascertain:

Is patient aware that control is poor and if so what changes have been implemented.

Has the patient had formal education ie seen a dietician, nurse specialist? Does the patient have access to a diabetic clinic?

Cardiac risks (family history, smoking, hypertension)

Past medical history

Family history of diabetes, hypertension

Current medication (remember that GP letters don't always state this)

Advice on possible causes of blurry vision, (lens shape alteration due to hyperglycaemia) but recommendation of eye check.

Possible amyotrophy.

Importance of good glycaemic control

Reference to UKPDS (United Kingdom Prospective Diabetes Study)

3.4.4 Tutorial: UKPDS

Patients with type 2 diabetes have excessive mortality from macrovascular disease (>70%). This group of patients are insulin resistant and are hence more prone to develop hypertension and dyslipidaemia which may be present in up to 50% of cases at the time of diagnosis and affect 70% or more after 15 years.

The UKPDS has been the largest and longest study to date on patients with type 2 diabetes. The study consisted of 5102 patients with newly diagnosed type 2 diabetes in 23 centres within the UK from 1977-1991. The patients were followed up for an average of 10 years in order to determine:

- Whether intensive pharmacological therapy to lower blood glucose levels would improve clinical outcomes, in particular a reduction in both macrovascular and microvascular disease.

- Whether there were any specific therapeutic advantages or disadvantages of using sulphonylureas, biguanides or insulin.

Furthermore patients who were also found to be hypertensive were randomised into 2 groups where one group were maintained with tight BP control (<145/85) and the other group lesser control to:

- Ascertain the benefits of lowering blood pressure in patients with type 2 diabetes

- To assess any advantages or disadvantages in using β blockers or ACE inhibitors.

Summary of the main conclusions of the UKPDS:

- 35% reduction of microvascular complications (retinopathy, nephropathy and possibly neuropathy) on lowering blood glucose levels in **intensive therapy** (HbA1 7%) compared to **conventional therapy** (HbA1 7.9%). This highlights that only a slight reduction in the HbA1 can have a tremendous impact on clinical outcome.

- There was no evidence of any glycaemic threshold for any of the microvascular complications above normal glucose levels (HbA1 >6.2).

- There was no significant effect of lowering blood glucose on macrovascular disease. There was a 16% reduction in the risk of combined fatal and non-fatal myocardial infarction which was not statistically significant. (p = 0.052). Epidemiological analysis did however show that for each %age reduction in the HbA1, there was:
  - 25% reduction in diabetes related deaths
  - 18% reduction in combined fatal and non-fatal MI
  - 7% reduction in all-cause mortality

- Again, there was no evidence of any glycaemic threshold for any of the microvascular complications above normal glucose levels (HbA1 >6.2).

- The highest average annual incidence of major hypoglycaemic events was 2.3% of patients per year in those receiving insulin therapy.

- The study showed that lowering the blood pressure to a mean of 144/82 mmHg significantly reduced :
    - Strokes
    - Diabetes related deaths
    - Heart failure
    - Microvascular complications
    - Visual loss

- Metformin: In this study obese patients were treated with metformin as well as other intensive and conventional therapies. In patients initially assigned to intensive therapy with metformin had a reduction in the following when compared to the conventionally treated patients.
    - Combined diabetes related end points
    - Diabetes related deaths
    - All cause deaths
    - Myocardial infarction

3.5 Case 5

3.5.1 Candidate information

Dear Doctor

This 36 year- old woman was recently started on warfarin for life. She was born with an atrial septal defect, which was corrected at the age of 34.

Since then she has been troubled intermittently by vague chest pains which have resulted in several hospital admissions. None of these has ever confirmed a myocardial infarction and a recent exercise test was inconclusive due to fatigue of the patient. An angiogram showed no significant pathology.

During her last admission 3 months ago she was found to be in fast atrial fibrillation. She has since been very anxious as her withdrawal bleeds from her HRT are more severe.

Thank you,

Dr Royle

Instructions to the candidate
You have 14 minutes with the patient and 1 minute for reflection before discussion with the examiners.

Take as detailed a general medical history as possible with emphasis on the cause for complaint

You are not expected to examine the patient.

Case 5

3.5.2 Subject Information

You are a 38 year old woman who was found to have a murmur during childhood.

You had no problems until your pregnancy 3 years ago when you became very breathless and were advised to have corrective heart surgery.

You had a premature menopause. You have been on HRT ever since without problems.

You have had stabbing chest pains which are associated with breathlessness ever since your cardiac surgery. You have been admitted to hospital from casualty 4 times with chest pain.

You are frustrated that your symptoms are still unaccountable.

You had an exercise test 6 months ago but got very breathless and it was stopped.

You then had a coronary angiogram which was essentially normal.

Three months ago you had palpitations and severe breathlessness.

You were found to have an irregular pulse and have since been started on warfarin.

You have noticed that this has made your withdrawal bleed from your HRT very heavy.

You are taking warfarin 4 mg a day and digoxin 500 mcg twice a day.

You have no allergies and no family history of disease.

You work as a nurse and are a non-smoker.

Case 5

3.5.3 Examiner information

In this scenario, the patient is clearly anxious and will lead the direction of history taking.

It tests the candidates ability to deal with a common problem which may be alarming simply because of the artificial exam set up.

This lady may be breathless for a number of reasons including atrial fibrillation, pulmonary hypertension, anaemia due to menorrhagia. She has had a premature menopause hence anaemia in this case may be caused by another autoimmune condition such as coeliacs.

In essence however, she has an ASD complicated by AF and Possibly pulmonary hypertension. The candidate will need to demonstrate that there is a definite connection here.

She has a normal angiogram but there has been no mention of an echocardiogram and the candidate will need to enquire specifically about this.

Topics for discussion:
- Indications for anticoagulation (atrial fibrillation, and risk of vascular accidents).
- Action of Warfarin: It inhibits the reductase enzyme responsible for regenerating the active form of vitamin K, thus producing effective vitamin K deficiency.
- Monitoring of INR (International Normalised Ratio)
- Drug interactions
- Contraindications: Peptic ulcer, bleeding disorders, cerebral aneurysms, endocarditis, severe hypertension, liver failure
- Informing all medical and dental staff about the drug especially prior to dental extraction.

3.5.4 Tutorial: Atrial septal defect

Atrial Septal Defect (ASD) is the most common congenital lesion in adults after bicuspid aortic valve. Whist the defect is often asymptomatic until adulthood. The three abnormalities consist of Ostium primum, secundum and sinus venosus.

Complications of an undetected lesion include:
- Pulmonary hypertension
- Right ventricular failure
- Atrial arrhythmias
- Paradoxical embolisation
- Cerebral abscess

- Although most cases are isolated , some individuals have a family history of this defect or other congenital cardiac abnormalities.
- Most patients with ASD with significant shunt flow (ie pulmonary to systemic flow more than 2:1) will be symptomatic by the age of 40. Atrial arrhythmia's, exercise intolerance, dyspnoea and fatigue are common in such patients and atrial arrhythmia's may be the most frequent presenting symptom in previously asymptomatic adults.
- Cardiac disease: atrial arrhythmia's increase with age and pulmonary artery pressure.
- Patients can develop stroke due to paradoxical embolization from a right to left shunt.
- The incidence of migraines is increased in patients with right to left shunts.
- Eisenmengers: This syndrome is characterised by the development of irreversible pulmonary hypertension at near systemic levels and reversal of shunt flow to a predominately right to left direction leading to cyanosis. The presence of moderate to severe pulmonary hypertension complicates less than 10% of cases at the time of diagnosis. Patients with a sinus venosus defect have higher pulmonary artery pressures and develop pulmonary hypertension at an earlier age compared to patients with other forms of ASD. The prognosis is poor once Eisenmengers develops with a total life expectancy usually considered to be less than 3 years.

Evaluation:
- Transthoracic imaging and an M-mode echocardiogram frequently provides the first confirmation of the diagnosis of ASD. The defect is best seen in the apical 4 chamber view in which the interatrial septum is parallel to the ultrasound beam. Visualisation may however be suboptimal particularly in obese subjects.
- Contrast echocardiography is useful to assess shunting. In a patent foramen ovale the flow is from right to left by definition. There may also be a transient reversal of flow through an uncomplicated foramen when the right sided pressure is increased e.g. with Valsalva maneuver or briefly during onset of left ventricular contraction. In ASD complicated by pulmonary hypertension the left to right shunt is reversed.
- Doppler flow echocardiography: The size of the ASD on 2D echocardiography does not correlate well with shunt flow measured at catheterization. Colour flow can be of use to confirm the presence of ASD and can be used to estimate the defect size but there are again limitations.
- Transesophageal echocardiography (TOE) is superior to transthoracic echocardiography in its ability to image the interatrial septum and is extremely accurate in the diagnosis of all three types of defects.

3.5.5 Tutorial: Warfarin

• The anticoagulant effect of is mediated by interference with the vitamin K-dependent gamma-carboxylation of coagulation factors II, VII, IX, and X, and proteins C and S]. This results in the synthesis of immunologically detectable but biologically inactive forms of these coagulation proteins.

• LABORATORY MONITORING and the INR: The laboratory test most commonly used to measure the effects of warfarin is the one-stage prothrombin time (PT) test. The PT is sensitive to reduced activity of factors II, VII, and X but is insensitive to reduced activity of factor IX. Confusion about the appropriate therapeutic range has occurred because the different tissue thromboplastins used for measuring the PT vary considerably in sensitivity to the vitamin K-dependent clotting factors and in response to warfarin].

• In order to promote standardization of the PT for monitoring oral anticoagulant therapy, the World Health Organization (WHO) developed an international reference thromboplastin from human brain tissue and recommended that the PT ratio be expressed as the International Normalized Ratio or INR].

• Initial dose and therapeutic range —Warfarin is administered in an initial dose of 5 to 10 mg per day for the first two days, with daily dose then adjusted according to the INR]. The desired INR varies with the clinical state, ranging from 2.0 to 3.0 in venous thromboembolism to 3.0 to 4.5 in patients with mechanical heart valves.

• The initiation of therapy with large loading doses has several potential complications, including excess anticoagulation and a transient hypercoagulable state due to a precipitous decline in protein C levels in first 36 hours.

• Loading is however necessary to allow for the delay until the normal clotting factors are cleared from the circulation and the peak effect does not occur until 36 to 72 hours after drug administration. During the first few days of warfarin therapy, the prolongation of the prothrombin time (PT) mainly reflects the depression of factor VII, which has a half-life of five to seven hours. This does not represent adequate anticoagulation, because the intrinsic and common clotting pathways remain intact until factors II, IX, and X are sufficiently reduced, which takes about five days with adequate dosing.

• Warfarin is the long-term anticoagulant of choice in nonpregnant patients, but its great disadvantage in pregnancy is that it freely crosses the placental barrier because of its low molecular weight and can harm the fetus. However, nursing mothers can safely take the drug because there is no convincing evidence that warfarin exerts an anticoagulant effect on the breast-fed infant.

• Adverse fetal effects from Warfarin may result from the teratogenicity of the drug and its propensity to cause bleeding in the fetus.
There is convincing evidence that Warfarin administration between the sixth and ninth weeks of gestation is potentially teratogenic]. The most common developmental abnormalities affect bone and cartilage; these simulate chondromalacia punctata, with stippled epiphyses and nasal and limb hypoplasia [The mechanism of this type of warfarin teratogenicity has not been established, but may be related to the drug's interference with the post-translational modification of calcium-binding proteins that are important for the normal growth and development of bony structures]. As an example, osteocalcin carboxylation

in human subjects is a vitamin K-dependent process, and circulating osteocalcin is structurally altered by warfarin. When used during the second and third trimesters of pregnancy, Warfarin has been linked to abnormalities of the fetal central nervous system, including optic atrophy, microcephaly, mental retardation, spasticity, and hypotonia. These central nervous system abnormalities are thought to be due to repeated cerebral micro hemorrhages, and may not be overt at birth .

- Clinicians are occasionally faced with the dilemma of managing pregnant patients who require ongoing anticoagulation for the prophylaxis or treatment of thrombotic complications. Examples include women with mechanical heart valves, venous thromboembolism immediately prior to or during pregnancy, severe congestive heart failure, and symptomatic antiphospholipid antibody syndrome. Strategies to maintain therapeutic anticoagulation while avoiding maternal or fetal harm due to antithrombotic agents are based largely upon retrospective data because ethical and legal considerations make large prospective trials among pregnant women difficult to conduct.

3.6 Case 6

3.6.1 Candidate information

Dear Doctor,

Thank you for seeing this 36 year old man who works as a security guard at the local fire station.

He has had two generalised seizures which have been witnessed by a neighbour on the first occasion, and the second by his colleagues at work following a night shift.

On the latter occasion, he sustained marked soft tissue bruising.

I did send him along to casualty but he was post-ictal and self-discharged prior to being assessed.

I would be grateful for your advice.

With best wishes

Dr Smith

Instructions to the candidate

You have 14 minutes with the patient and 1 minute for reflection before discussion with the examiners.

Take as detailed a general medical history as possible with emphasis on the cause for complaint

You are not expected to examine the patient.

Case 6

3.6.2 Subject Information

Alcoholic liver disease with generalised seizures due to acute withdrawal.

You are a 36 year old single man.

You have moved to London from Scotland 2 years ago after finishing your degree in History.

You would like to work in a museum but have not managed to find the type of work you like.

You live alone and have no real friends although your neighbours are friendly. You had made friends but have fallen out with most of them, (eventually admit that it was because of your drinking habits).

You have been working as a security guard doing nights because you can't find other work.

You have been drinking alcohol to help you sleep during the day.

You drink on average 2 bottles of red wine during the day but for the last 2 months have been brewing your own beer as it is cheaper.

You wake up every 2-3 hours during the day and have a drink.

You have noticed that your hands shake during the night when you are at work and feel that you have problems speaking to people unless you have had a drink because you feel shy.

You have been told that you have had 2 fits but cannot remember anything about them other than bruising your back and biting into your cheek. You have also had a lot of pain below your right ribs and have been told by your GP that the liver is enlarged. The fits occurred at a time when you were trying to give up drinking.

You do not smoke.

Your father died at the age of 54 (3 years ago) after a fall, which resulted in a brain haemorrhage. He was an alcoholic. Your mother has gout and a high blood pressure. Your GP has started you on vitamin tablets and advised you to reduce your alcohol intake. You have also been given some diazepam to help you sleep.

Case 6

3.6.3 Examiner Information
Alcoholic liver disease with generalised seizures due to acute alcohol withdrawal.
This is a young man with a multitude of problems that occur as a result of social isolation. He has moved to a new town, works nights and sleeps in the day and has no friends.

He is intelligent in that he has a degree and he also has ambitions to work in a museum.

His alcohol intake is excessive and he drinks alone.

He has been in denial.

The candidate should ask the CAGE / Control questions.
- Can you always **co**ntrol your drinking?
- Has alcohol ever led you to **n**eglect your family or your work?
- What **t**ime do you start drinking?
- Have your friends or family ever commented that you should **r**educe your intake?
- Do you ever drink in the mornings to **o**vercome a hangover?
- Go through an average day's alcohol intake **l**eaving nothing out.

Suicide risk should also be addressed.

3.6.4 Tutorial: Alcohol Withdrawal Symptoms
- It is not entirely clear why some individuals suffer from more severe withdrawal symptoms than others. Experiments in 1955 demonstrated that people who drank for 7 to 34 consecutive days developed minor withdrawal symptoms upon cessation of alcohol, while drinking for 48 to 87 consecutive days resulted in major withdrawal symptoms in 5 of 6 subjects. These results imply that most people are vulnerable to the effects of the abrupt cessation of prolonged, sustained ethanol intake.

- Symptoms of alcohol withdrawal occur because alcohol is a central nervous system depressant; abrupt withdrawal unmasks compensatory over activity of certain parts of the nervous system, including sympathetic autonomic outflow. Altered levels of several neurotransmitters have been noted, and may be important in the pathophysiology of alcohol withdrawal:

- Gamma-aminobutyric acid (GABA) is the major inhibitory neurotransmitter in the brain. Its receptor is down regulated and its neuronal activity decreased in alcohol withdrawal, resulting in hyperarousal.

- Elevated levels of Noradrenaline are found in the cerebrospinal fluid of patients withdrawing from alcohol and are believed due to a decrease in the alpha-2 receptor-mediated inhibition of presynaptic norepinephrine release]. This may explain some reported benefits of clonidine which potentiates alpha-2 receptor activity in the brain.

- Serotonin and its degradation products have been implicated in both tolerance and craving for alcohol. Similarly, some of the by-products of alcohol metabolism, such as acetaldehyde, have been shown to enhance subjects' "appetite" for alcohol and may contribute to their addiction.

<u>Minor withdrawal symptoms:</u>

Minor withdrawal symptoms are due to central nervous system and sympathetic hyperactivity, and can include insomnia, tremor, mild anxiety, gastrointestinal upset, headache, diaphoresis, palpitations, or anorexia. Symptoms usually are present within six hours of the cessation of drinking and may develop while patients still have a significant alcohol level in their blood Findings resolve within 24 to 48 hours. The specific minor withdrawal symptoms in a given patient typically are consistent from one episode to the next.

WITHDRAWAL SEIZURES

Withdrawal seizures are generalized tonic-clonic convulsions usually occurring within 48 hours after the last drink, and may occur after only 2 hours of abstinence. Approximately 3% of chronic alcoholics have withdrawal-associated seizures and, of those patients, 3% develop status epilepticus. Withdrawal seizures are predominantly seen in patients with a long history of chronic alcoholism.

ALCOHOLIC HALLUCINOSIS

Despite a tendency to equate alcoholic hallucinosis with delirium tremens, the two are not synonymous. Alcoholic hallucinosis refers to hallucinations which develop within 12 to 24 hours of abstinence and resolve within 24 to 48 hours (which is the earliest point at which delirium tremens typically develops). Hallucinations are usually visual, although auditory and tactile phenomena may also occur. In contrast to delirium tremens, alcoholic hallucinosis is not associated with global clouding of the senses but rather with specific hallucinations.

DELIRIUM TREMENS

Approximately 5% of patients who undergo withdrawal from alcohol suffer from delirium tremens (DTs), a syndrome characterized by hallucinations, disorientation, tachycardia, hypertension, low grade fever, agitation, and diaphoresis. DTs typically begin between 48 and 96 hours after the last drink and last 1 to 5 days.

Risk factors for the development of DTs include:
- A history of sustained drinking
- A history of previous DTs
- Age greater than 30
- The presence of a concurrent illness
- A greater number of days since the last drink (for example, patients who present more than two days after their last drink for treatment of alcohol withdrawal are more likely to experience DTs than those who present within two days)

The condition is associated with a mortality rate of up to 5%. Death usually is due to arrhythmias or complicating illnesses such as pneumonia. Older age, pre-existing pulmonary disease, core body temperature greater than 104°F, and coexisting liver disease are associated with a greater risk of mortality.

Clinical manifestations: DTs generally produce hallucinations, disorientation, tachycardia, hypertension, low grade fever, agitation, and diaphoresis. Patients with DTs have significantly elevated cardiac indices, oxygen delivery, and oxygen consumption. Arterial pH rises due to hyperventilation, which may be a rebound effect related to the respiratory depressant properties of alcohol. Hyperventilation and consequent respiratory alkalosis in this setting result in a significant decrease in cerebral blood flow. There is a correlation between the length of the preceding alcohol binge, the degree cerebral compromise, and the average %age reduction cerebral blood flow in patients with DTs, although there is no association between blood flow parameters and hallucinations or tremors.

Withdrawal may also have an important impact on fluid and electrolyte status. Almost all patients in acute withdrawal are dehydrated as a result of diaphoresis, hyperthermia, vomiting, and tachypnea. Hypokalemia is common due to renal and extra-renal losses, alterations in aldosterone levels, and changes in potassium distribution across the cell membrane. Hypomagnesemia occurs frequently with DTs and may predispose to withdrawal seizures. Hypophosphatemia may occur due to malnutrition, may be symptomatic, and if severe, may contribute to cardiac failure and rhabdomyolysis.

TREATMENT: Frequent evaluation of the patient and the avoidance of complacency are paramount in the management of alcohol withdrawal. Withdrawal syndromes may coexist with, or be mimicked by other conditions such as infection, trauma, metabolic derangements, drug overdose, hepatic failure, or gastrointestinal bleeding. Withdrawal is a diagnosis of exclusion, and it may be necessary to perform extensive testing, such as lumbar puncture and CT scan, to confidently exclude other diagnostic considerations, especially when patients present with an altered mental status and fever.

Once comorbid illnesses have been excluded or adequately treated, the management of alcohol withdrawal is directed at alleviating the symptoms and identifying and correcting metabolic derangements. Patients should be placed in a quiet, protective environment. Mechanical restraints with the patient in the lateral decubitus (or "swimmer's") position is usually necessary for patients suffering from DTs for the protection of both the patient and his caretakers. Volume deficits can be calculated and replaced accordingly or, if there are no contraindications, isotonic intravenous fluid can be infused rapidly until patients are clinically euvolemic.

Thiamine 100 mg IV or IM, should be administered prior to any glucose-containing solutions in order to decrease the risk of precipitating Wernicke's encephalopathy or Korsakoff's syndrome. Multivitamins containing or supplemented with folate should be given routinely, and deficiencies of potassium, magnesium, glucose, and phosphate should be corrected as needed. Patients considered to be at high risk for complications should be monitored in a high dependency or intensive care unit.

Benzodiazepines: Benzodiazepines are used to treat the psychomotor agitation most patients experience during withdrawal and to prevent progression from minor withdrawal symptoms to major ones].Chlordiazepoxide and Diazepam are used most frequently to treat or prevent alcohol withdrawal, but other benzodiazepine agents also can be used. In general, long-acting agents are preferred because they seem to result in a smoother course with less chance of recurrent withdrawal or seizures. Oxazepam and Lorazepam are minimally metabolized in the liver and may be useful in the treatment of patients with cirrhosis, while agents which are available in parenteral form (e.g., lorazepam, diazepam) may be necessary in patients who cannot receive oral medications.

Titration of medications should be based upon a given patient's risk factors for and ability to tolerate DTs. As an example, a patient younger than 45 years old with no other illnesses should be lightly sedated to insure his safety and comfort but allow his neurological exam to be followed. In contrast, an older patient with pre-existing cardiopulmonary disease should be kept more heavily sedated and should be monitored in an intensive care unit because they are at greater risk and may not tolerate the systemic stress of major withdrawal.

3.7 Case 7

3.7.1 Candidate information

Dear Casualty Doctor,

Thank you for seeing this 35 year old man who has just returned from a 6 month visit to Thailand.

He has lost 5 stones in weight and has recently had a bout of chicken pox.

This did affect his lungs and I treated him for a chest infection with a course of antibiotics.

My main concern is that he still has a fever and complains of breathlessness six weeks later.

Please advise,

Kind regards

Doctor Bingham

Instructions to the candidate

You have 14 minutes with the patient and 1 minute for reflection before discussion with the examiners.

Take as detailed a general medical history as possible with emphasis on the cause for complaint

You are not expected to examine the patient.

Case 7

3.7.2 Subject information

You are a 30 year old Freelance journalist.

You tend to write about drug culture and music.

You have returned from a 6 month sabbatical in Thailand.

Shortly after arriving back to England, you developed chicken pox much to your amusement and annoyance.

You were told that it also affected your lungs but 6 weeks after the infection has cleared, you are still breathless and have fevers.

Symptoms:
Previously, you could run for several miles, but at present, can only walk briskly for 30-40 meters before you become breathless.

You have a dry irritating cough.

You have lost 5 stones in weight and feel a lot of this is loss of muscle mass because you can't exercise anymore.

You don't feel very hungry at the moment.

Your past history:

You had glandular fever 4 months ago whilst in Thailand. Otherwise you have only suffered from the usual childhood illnesses.

Social
You stopped smoking when you got chicken pox, but prior to this you smoked 10 cigarettes a day.

You have always been careful in your sexual practice and do not take drugs yourself, but you do have friends who are dependent on class A drugs.

You have had 6 sexual partners in the last year. You did have unprotected sex with a woman you met in Thailand 6 months ago and are still in contact with her. She worked as a dancer. Initially you were careful, but as you became closer, you realised that she was "all right" and became careless.

Case 7

3.7.3 Examiner Information:

Case: Breathlessness, query HIV infection.

This young man has had unprotected sex in a high risk area.

He developed glandular fever like symptoms shortly after this which could correspond to seroconversion.

He has since had chicken pox and what could be pneumocystis carinii infection reflecting immuno compromise.

Candidate:
- Should ascertain the extent of the symptoms and attribute a clear time scale in the events of deterioration.

- Must elicit a good social and sexual history

- Consider other complications and actively enquire about a general review of symptoms

- Establish any sexual partners since the return from Thailand

- Establish an investigation protocol

- Show empathy towards patient who at this stage has little insight into possible diagnosis.

3.7.4 Tutorial: Pneumocystis Carinii

Pneumocystis carinii pneumonia (PCP) is a life threatening opportunistic infection which occurs in immunocompromised hosts especially patients with HIV infection. This infection is also increasing in frequency in patients who are immunosuppressed such as organ transplant recipients, malignancy (more commonly haematological rather than solid tumours) and those treated with chemotherapeutic regimens.

EPIDEMIOLOGY: The organism is believed to be transmitted by the respiratory-aerosol route, and 75% of humans are infected by age four. These primary infections are probably asymptomatic. Although most cases of PCP are believed to represent reactivation of latent disease, there are animal data suggesting that animal to animal transmission is possible. Reports of cluster outbreaks in oncology units and among HIV-infected patients suggest that human to human transmission is possible, but genotypic analyses indicate that acquisition of infection in such a manner is relatively infrequent and accounts for a minority of cases.

The incidence of PCP in HIV-infected patients increases as the CD4 count decreases. Generally, PCP does not occur until the CD4 count drops below 200 cells/mm^3. In a study of over 1100 individuals with HIV infection, the Pulmonary Complications of HIV Infection Study Group confirmed the relationship between CD4 cell count and PCP. 95% of patients who developed PCP had a CD4 count below 200 cells/mm^3. HIV transmission category, age, smoking history, and use of antiretroviral therapy did not predict development of PCP; black subjects had one third the risk of PCP compared to white patients.

Clinical manifestations: In HIV-infected patients, PCP is generally gradual in onset and characterized by fever (79% to 100%), cough (95%), and progressive dyspnoea (95%). The cough is usually non-productive, but as many as 30% of patients may have some sputum production. Other symptoms include fatigue, rigors, chest pain, and weight loss. Approximately seven % of patients are asymptomatic.

Physical examination: The most common findings on physical examination are fever (84% of patients have a temperature exceeding 38.1°C) and tachypnea (62%). Respiratory auscultation may be normal but wheeze and crepitations may be audible in 50% of cases.

Extrapulmonary manifestations of P. carinii infection, such as hepatosplenomegaly, skin lesions, and pleural effusions, are increasing in part due to localized PCP prophylaxis with aerosolized pentamidine.

Radiographic manifestations:

The most common radiographic abnormalities are diffuse, bilateral interstitial or alveolar infiltrates. Although upper lobe infiltrates can be seen de novo, a higher incidence of predominantly apical infiltrates is reported in patients using aerosolized pentamidine prophylaxis]. Other, less common presentations include:

- Pneumothoraces
- Lobar or segmental infiltrates
- Cysts
- Nodules
- Pleural effusions

High resolution computed tomography (HRCT) has a high sensitivity for PCP among HIV-positive patients. One study, for example, evaluated 51 patients with suspected PCP and normal, equivocal, or nonspecific chest x-ray findings; HRCT had a sensitivity of 100 % and a specificity of 89 % when the presence of patchy or nodular ground-glass attenuation was used to indicate possible PCP. A negative HRCT may allow exclusion of PCP in such patients.

3.8 Case 8

3.8.1 Candidate information

You are the medical SHO covering casualty. You receive a referral from a local GP and agree to review the patient.

Dear doctor,

Thank you for seeing this 28 year old lady who has suffered 2 blackouts in the last 48 hours.

She has not had chest pains.

Her ECG is unremarkable.

Please advise.

Doctor Carr.

Instructions to the candidate

You have 14 minutes with the patient and 1 minute for reflection before discussion with the examiners.

Take as detailed a general medical history as possible with emphasis on the cause for complaint

You are not expected to examine the patient.

Case 8

3.8.2 Subject Information:

You are a 28 year old dance teacher.

Problem: You have had 2 distinct lapses in your memory where you feel that you may have had a blackout.

Yesterday in the afternoon, you were lying on the sofa and speaking to your mother on the phone but cannot remember the conversation.

At one moment you were speaking to her and the next you notice the phone receiver is on the floor. You are not hurt but felt vague for several hours after that.

You convinced yourself that you had probably fallen asleep.

Today whilst having lunch with your boyfriend and his parents, they claim that you became totally vacant and you dropped your cutlery. Your boyfriend thinks that your fingers twitched a little. You felt vague after this but don't feel too bad now.

Your boyfriends mum is a nurse and she suggested that you go to casualty.

You have been previously well.

You currently take the oral contraceptive.

You have recently been treated for a urinary tract infection (you have just completed your antibiotic course).

You smoke 10 cigarettes a day.

You live with your boyfriend.

You drink 2 glasses of white wine most evenings.

Your brother was diagnosed of suffering from epilepsy at the age of 7 but has not had a problem as far as you are concerned for many years.

Case 8

3.8.3 Examiner information:

Case: Blackouts query cause.

The likely diagnosis is petit mal seizures although one cannot and must not assume this as the only diagnosis.

- In the presenting complaint, the candidate should have explored all aspects from the presenting complaint including neurological, cardiac and hyperventilatory symptoms.

- This includes headaches, dizziness, palpitations, perioral paraesthesia

- As much detail should be gathered about the patients degree of alertness after the event.

- In adult onset epilepsy, care must be taken to search for and exclude a structural pathology. The candidate should establish this by actively asking about any history of previous head injury or birth trauma, symptoms of cerebral space occupying lesion such as headaches, past history of hypertension, alcohol intake.

- Drug history including recreational drugs

The candidate should be expected to be competent in investigating this patient with

- U&E, LFT's, glucose, Ca2+, PO4, serum and urine toxic screens

- CT brain & EEG

3.9 Case 9

3.9.1 Candidate information

You are the medical SHO seeing a patient in the general medical clinic.

Dear Doctor,

Thank you for seeing this 26 year old lady who has been troubled by loose stools admixed with blood.

On examination her abdomen was soft but tender on deep palpation in the left iliac fossa.

Her haemoglobin is 8.5 with a microcytic picture.

I would be grateful for your hasty assessment.

Thank you kindly

Dr Hall

Instructions to the candidate

You have 14 minutes with the patient and 1 minute for reflection before discussion with the examiners.

Take as detailed a general medical history as possible with emphasis on the cause for complaint

You are not expected to examine the patient.

Case 9

3.9.2 Subject information

You are a 28 year old actress.

You have noticed a gradual onset of loose motions over the last 8 months.

Previously you opened your bowels once a day usually first thing in the morning.

You first noticed that your motions became loose and you were going 2-3 times a day. The stool was soft and you did not notice any blood in it although you were not actively looking at it! At this time, you initially felt unwell and lost your appetite for a few weeks but then things settled down over the next few months.

2 months ago, the symptoms recurred but this time the soft stool has progressed to frank diarrhoea. You can open you bowels from 6-10 times a day. To your horror, you have noticed blood which is both bright red and dark in the stool. There appears to be quite a lot of it. Your stools are also slimy now and often when you have finished, you feel like you still want to go. You may at this time pass just blood or mucus if you strain.

You feel unwell and have lost over a stone in weight. You feel a little hot and sweaty.

You have intermittently suffered from mouth ulcers in the last 4 years but just use an antibacterial mouth wash.

You past medical history is a healthy one.

You have suffered from low back pain but think it may be caused by your posture.

You stopped smoking a year ago.

You are a social drinker, consuming 2-4 units a week (if at all).

You have never been abroad.

You are a vegetarian.

Case 9

3.9.3 Examiner Information

Case: Bloody diarrhoea

The differential diagnosis here is inflammatory bowel disease.
*   The candidate should ascertain the gradual onset of symptoms which would make food poisoning unlikely

*   A clear account should be taken as to what the patient actually means by diarrhoea

*   The candidate should be able to elicit that there is blood and mucus in the stools as well as symptoms of tenesmus

*   Systemic symptoms such as anorexia, malaise should be sort after

*   The candidate should also exclude symptoms that indicate an acute exacerbation such as abdominal pain, fever, tachycardia and abdominal distension.

*   Ascertain the severity attributed to the symptoms

Points for discussion
*   The differential diagnosis (UC/ Crohn's)
*   Complications of UC
*   Investigation: Bloods, colonoscopy/ sigmoidoscopy, rectal biopsy
*   Management

3.10 Case 10
3.10.1 Candidate information

You are the medical SHO seeing a patient in the general medical clinic.

Dear Doctor,

This 70 year old man has had a tremor in his hands for 4 months. It is gradually getting worse and he is quite embarrassed by it when he is in company. The tremor is worse in his right hand. He sometimes gets tremors in his legs.

He retired 5 years ago from his job as a postman. He is quite anxious and is starting to wonder if there is something seriously wrong,

Thank you,

Yours Sincerely,

Dr. Walsh

Instructions to the candidate

You have 14 minutes with the patient and 1 minute for reflection before discussion with the examiners.

Take as detailed a general medical history as possible with emphasis on the cause for complaint

You are not expected to examine the patient.

Case 10

3.10.2   Subject information

You are a 70-year-old man with a tremor. The tremor is in both hands and has been present for 4 months. It is gradually getting worse and you are quite embarrassed by it when in company. The tremor is worse in your right hand. You sometimes get tremors in your legs.

The tremor is present when you are doing nothing and tends to disappear when you move your hands - to drink from a cup for example. You are also quite stiff around your shoulders especially in the mornings. Your speech is normal but some people have commented that your handwriting has gotten smaller over the years. Your walking has got slower but you think that this may be due to old age. Sometimes you get dizzy when you stand up too quickly. There is no family history of anyone with a tremor.

You drink about 2 pints of beer per week – drinking has no effect on the tremor. You smoke about 10 cigarettes a day. You feel down at times as you are worried about the tremor. Your memory is perfect.

You have had no previous illnesses and you take no medications. You have never had a head injury.

You retired 5 years ago from your job as a postman. You are quite anxious about the tremor and are starting to wonder if there is something seriously wrong.

Case 10

3.10.3 Examiner information

Case: Parkinson's disease

This scenario tests the candidate's ability to take a history from a patient with a tremor.

The history points to a diagnosis of Parkinson's disease (PD). The candidate should demonstrate this by asking questions to draw out the following points:

➢ The tremor is in the hands and also slightly in the legs – this is typical of PD
➢ PD is typically worse on one side or the other
➢ The tremor is resting - this is typical of PD
➢ The patient is stiff – this may be the start of rigidity
➢ The gait is slow – the candidate should also ask if the patient has trouble turning around or if they have stopped swinging their arms or if they tend to get stuck at doorways – these are typical of PD
➢ The patient has micrographia

The candidate should also ask about
➢ Akinesia ("has anyone ever commented that your face seems to be blank?")
➢ Speech (typically low in volume)
➢ Swallowing (may be affected in advanced PD)
➢ Mood – often low in PD
➢ Memory – often impaired in advanced PD (this is due to Lewy body dementia)
➢ Falls
➢ Constipation

The candidate should rule out other common causes of tremor – for example the lack of family history and the fact that alcohol has no effect on the tremor virtually rules out the diagnosis of essential tremor. The candidate should also ask about other symptoms of hyperthyroidism beside tremor.

The candidate should also ask what effect the tremor is having on the patient's life: they should take a good social history and should also ask about driving. The candidate should also ask about occupation (farmers have an increased risk of PD possible because they are exposed to insecticides).

The excellent candidate will seek out the cause of the parkinsonism: is it idiopathic PD or is there another cause?
➢ drug induced parkinsonism (the candidate should ask about antipsychotic and antinausea drugs)
➢ head trauma
➢ vascular pseudo-parkinsonism (any history of strokes or hypertension)
➢ encephalitis
➢ Progressive supranuclear palsy (any double vision on looking upwards)
➢ Multisystem atrophy (formerly called Shy Drager syndrome): this is characterised by parkinsonism, postural hypotension, urinary incontinence and impotence

However you should remember that postural hypotension can be a feature of idiopathic PD and can be caused by drugs used to treat PD (e.g. levodopa and the dopamine agonists).

NB: Most patients with tremors are embarrassed by their tremor: this does not point to a particular diagnosis.

Case 10

3.10.4   Tutorial: Parkinson's disease

Parkinson's disease is a common disorder that affects men and women approximately equally. It occurs in all ethnic groups and becomes increasingly common in old age.

Diagnosis

The core clinical features are
- Resting tremor
- Paucity of movement
- Slow movement
- Cog wheel rigidity
- Postural instability.

The tremor is typically worse on one side or the other in early PD until as the disease advances it becomes more generalised. Another core feature of PD is a clear response to dopaminergic medication. The gait is typically slow and the patient often has trouble turning around or has lost their arm swing. Sometimes they get stuck in doorways and as the disease advances they can fall over.

Other features of PD include
- micrographia
- low volume speech
- impaired swallowing in advanced PD
- low mood
- impaired memory (this is due to Lewy body dementia)
- constipation

Differential diagnosis

This includes
- drug induced parkinsonism
- head trauma
- vascular pseudo parkinsonism
- Progressive supranuclear palsy (parkinsonism, upward gaze palsy, and axial dystonia)
- Cortico basal ganglionic degeneration (parkinsonism, apraxia, sensory inattention, dementia, aphasia)
- Multisystem atrophy (formerly called Shy Drager syndrome): this is characterised by parkinsonism, postural hypotension, urinary incontinence and impotence

However you should remember that postural hypotension can be a feature of idiopathic PD and can be caused by drugs used to treat PD (e.g. levodopa and the dopamine agonists).

More rare differentials include
- Wilson's disease (young onset, chronic hepatitis, Kayser-Fleischer rings)
- Huntingdon's disease (chorea, autosomal dominant inheritance, early onset dementia)
- Creutzfeldt Jacob disease (myoclonus, ataxia, early onset dementia)

Treatment
Drug treatment is not always needed early in the course of disease. Patients should be started on drug treatment when the disease has started to affect their everyday life.

Levodopa
This is still the mainstay of drug treatment. It helps all the major symptoms of PD but does not slow the progression of the disease. Short term side effects include nausea and vomiting and postural hypotension. Dyskinesias, the on-off phenomena and end of dose fluctuations occur later on in the course of treatment. Levodopa is given in combination with carbidopa which is a dopa decarboxylase inhibitor that inhibits the peripheral breakdown of levodopa thus allowing more levodopa to get into the central nervous system.

Dopamine agonists
Dopamine agonist act directly on the dopamine receptors in the CNS. Their use is associated with a lower risk of dyskinesias than with levodopa. Side effects include nausea and vomiting and postural hypotension. Their use is probably associated with a higher risk of psychotic symptoms than that seen with levodopa.

COMT inhibitors
Catechol-O-methyl transferase inhibitors block the breakdown of levodopa and thus help to smooth out dyskinesias associated with the use of levodopa. Entacapone is the only COMT inhibitor licensed for use in the UK.

Selegiline
This is a mono-amine oxidase inhibitor type B. It inhibits the breakdown of dopamine and thus helps parkinsonian symptoms. There were hopes that selegiline would delay the progression of the disease but these hopes have now largely foundered.
Anticholinergic drugs

These can help tremor and rigidity but they cause a range of side effects such as dry mouth, nausea, constipation urinary retention and confusion. They are often poorly tolerated by people with Parkinson's disease and particularly by elderly patients

General measures
Physiotherapy and occupational therapy and speech therapy can help parkinsonian symptoms and can help patients to live as normal a life as possible.

Surgery
Thalamotomy and pallidotomy can help some patients who no longer respond to medical treatment. But these forms of neurosurgery can cause a range of complications and should only be used a last resort.

Deep brain stimulation
High-frequency stimulation of the subthalamic nuclei or globus pallidus can help to alleviate parkinsonian symptoms. Unlike surgery this treatment is reversible and it is being increasingly explored in patients who no longer respond to medication or have intolerable side effects from medication.

3.11 Case 11

3.11.1 Candidate information

Dear Doctor

Re: Douglas Pouch

Thank you for reviewing this 56-year-old builder, who is troubled with difficulty in breathing.

He was seen in your Casualty Department two weeks ago and started on inhalers.

Unfortunately, he is rather overweight with a BMI of 32 and smokes six cigarettes a day. I have offered him advice on smoking cessation and I will be grateful for your further investigations.

His peak flow in my Clinic was 130 L/minute this afternoon.

Yours sincerely

Dr French

You have 14 minutes with the patient and 1 minute for reflection before discussion with the examiners.

Take as detailed a general medical history as possible with emphasis on the cause for complaint

You are not expected to examine the patient.

Case 11

3.11.2   Subject information

You are a 56-year-old man who has worked as builder since the age of 18. You are always very active and although you do less building now, you actually manage a small building company that deals with contracts throughout the area. In your early days as a builder, you did work on demolition of an old hospital and an old school, where there was a danger of asbestos threatening the community. You were not, at that time, aware of any dangers. You have been becoming gradually short of breath, for the last six years.

You first noticed it during the summer holidays in Malta, when you felt breathless and wheezy in the first week of your holiday. You saw a local Doctor who prescribed antibiotics and you were able to enjoy the last week of your holiday there. You hardly ever go to the Doctors. A month ago you started feeling breathless at rest and on exertion. You tried to ignore it and felt that you might just have a minor chest infection, but two weeks later you were taken to A&E by your son, who became very concerned by your wheezing. Your son thought that you looked blue. In casualty you had been given a nebuliser and a steroid injection and it was thought that you were well enough to leave after a few hours. You have been troubled by cough for the last five or six years and tend to cough up sputum most mornings. You have not been troubled by any chest pain or ankle swellings. You have never coughed up any blood or had any skin rashes.

When you were younger you smoked 40 cigarettes a day but cut this down to about six, six years ago. You drink two pints of beer a day, but have stopped this, since you have not felt so well. You were very concerned as the inhalers given to you by the Casualty have not made much difference to your symptoms and you feel that if anything you are getting worse.

Case 11

3.11.3   Examiner information

A good candidate will be able to elicit that this gentleman's respiratory symptoms occurred six years ago and did not trouble him until the last month. One should be taken to differentiate between breathlessness caused by ischaemic heart disease and that caused by intrinsic lung disease. Also, one should focus on a thorough occupational history, specific questions on asbestos and other forms of occupational lung disease. Questions should also be asked as to whether the subject has been immunized for tuberculosis and whether there are other symptoms of TB. A complete smoking history in terms of pack years should be ascertained. Detailed drug history including the use of drugs that cause lung fibrosis should be searched for. What investigations would the candidate, consider? Full blood count, urea electrolytes, chest x-ray, ECG, full lung function tests including spirometry, lung volume diffusion, flow volume loop reversibility and forced expiratory volume in one second.

3.12 Case 12

3.12.1 Candidate information

Dear Doctor

Re: Samantha Keates

I would be grateful for your assessment of this 24-year-old Jamaican lady who had been previously well until nine months ago. Since then she has suffered from intermittent fevers and did complain initially of dysuria. All of her MSU's have been negative. There has been no history of travel abroad and certainly no obvious infective focus.

In the last four months she has been troubled by intermittent diarrhoea. She has also developed an arthritis affecting her hands and her ankles. Her full blood count has shown a normochromic normocytic anaemia although her U+E's and LFT's are within normal limits. Her ESR was raised at 90.

I would be grateful for any further advice.

With best wishes.

Yours sincerely

Dr Katz

You have 14 minutes with the patient and 1 minute for reflection before discussion with the examiners.

Take as detailed a general medical history as possible with emphasis on the cause for complaint

You are not expected to examine the patient.

Case 12

3.12.2 Subject information

You are a 24-year-old secretary. You have always been well apart from a seizure that you suffered from at the age of 22. You were studying at college at the time and you were admitted to hospital where you were found to have a high temperature. You had been discharged the following day as you felt well. You were told that you would be sent a further appointment although nothing arrived, and as you felt better you did not follow things up.

In the last nine months you have had symptoms of feeling generally tired and under the weather although nothing specific. You have felt generally down in the dumps because you know that all is not well with your health. You have been to see the GP so many times, and whilst you know that you are not well you cannot be specific as your symptoms are so vague. You have suffered from diarrhoea and have lost weight. You have had several viral infections which have caused you difficulty in taking deep breaths in. These have tended to occur three times over the last nine months. You travel to work in the train and have attributed these to viral infections that you have picked up from fellow commuters.

You have also noticed weaknesses in the tops of your legs, which feel like jelly when you stand. You have always suffered from cold fingers for as long as you remember and your mother and grandmother also suffer from this. You always wear gloves in the winter. In the recent months you have found that you have been breathless although your GP thought initially that this might just be anxiety. You have noticed that you tend to develop weals on your skin and had a private appointment with a dermatologist, who reassured you that it was urticaria.

You consume two units of alcohol a week and do not smoke. You have never been abroad. You live at home with your partner, who is a teacher at a local secondary school, and your two-year-old son.

Case 12

3.12.3   Examiner information

Based on this history alone the candidate must really focus on excluding an infectious or autoimmune pathology. The patient is a young female Jamaican lady and for this reason a vigilant candidate of focus and eliciting further information that may suggest an underlying cause of a connective tissue disease. SLE is extremely variable in its manifestation although the fever is common and exacerbations occur in over 80% of patients. A candidate would question specifically for symptoms of malaise and fatigue. Joint involvement also occurs in over 90% of patients and may manifest in a rheumatoid arthritis pattern. Joint pain is typically severe although in early stages the joints may appear entirely normal. Myalgia is also common. The candidate would need to focus on skin disorders which occur in over 80% of cases, specifically symptoms such as photosensitivity or a butterfly rash. A history of Raynaud's phenomenon would be absolutely essential in this case.

The candidate would also want to ask if there had been any previous episodes of seizures or peripheral neuropathy. Less frequently the patient may have symptoms of lung disease presenting with recurrent pleurisy or pleural effusions resulting in shortness of breath. Cardiac involvement occurs in less than half of cases and a mild myocarditis is common. Endocarditis involving the mitral valve (Libman-Sacks syndrome is very rare). It is important to ask this lady if there has been a history of hypertension which, whilst common in her ethnicity may also be a result of renal involvement. It is also imperative to take a drug history to ensure that this is not a case of drug induced SLE.

The key features in the GP's letter suggest a normochromic normocytic anaemia and a raised ESR, which in this situation would be in proportion to the disease activity.

The candidate would need to be aware of further investigations such as antinuclear antibodies, which are positive in most cases. Double-stranded DNA binding is specific for SLE although it is only present in 50% of cases, particularly those with severe systemic involvement. Rheumatoid factor is positive in half of cases with SLE. Serum complement levels are reduced during active disease. CRP is **normal.** Immunoglobulins are raised, usually IgG and IgM. Immunofluorescence skin biopsies would demonstrate immunoglobulin and complement deposition at the dermo-epidermal junction. This is known as the positive band test.

The candidate must be able to discuss drug therapy in SLE, starting with the use of corticosteroid therapy which is the mainstay of treatment in SLE, although patients with mild disease and arthralgia can be managed with non-steroidal anti-inflammatory drugs. In active SLE we feel that in pleurisy the patient should be treated with Prednisolone 30 mg daily, reducing over three to four weeks to a maintenance level of 5-10 mg a day. It may be possible to discontinue the treatment after six to eight weeks.

Other drug therapies in SLE:

1. Anti-malarial drug Chloroquine is used for suppressing disease activity in patients with minor manifestations such as arthralgia which cannot be controlled with non-steroidal anti-inflammatory drugs.

2. Immunosuppressive drugs are used in patients with more serious disease manifestation such as established renal disease. These drugs include Azathioprine, Chlorambucil or Cyclophosphamide. The disease tends to run an episodic course with exacerbations and complete remissions which may last for up to years at a time.

Other useful tips: - it is also important that the candidate works to exclude other connective tissue diseases, particularly systemic sclerosis. A history of dysphagia must be thought of.

3.13 Case 13

3.13.1   Candidate Information

Dear Doctor

Re: Mrs Debbie Singh – age 40.

I would be grateful for your advice on this patient who presented to me with several months of headaches. The headaches are now occurring every day and she is taking an increasing amount of time off work. She is concerned that her job may be at risk unless the situation improves.

The patient has been reasonably fit over the years. Her only recent contact with the health centre has been for menorrhagia for which she has been referred to a gynaecologist.

She is increasingly worried about her headaches and is currently taking up to eight Co-codamol tablets per day.

I would be grateful for your advice on future management.

With best wishes.

Yours sincerely,

Dr Kalia

You have 14 minutes with the patient and 1 minute for reflection before discussion with the examiners.

Take as detailed a general medical history as possible with emphasis on the cause for complaint

You are not expected to examine the patient.

Case 13

3.13.2   Subject information:

History of presenting symptoms
You have been getting severe headaches which occur daily and, because of these, you have been taking a lot of sick leave from work. You work in an office as a secretary and your employer has made several comments about your sickness levels over the past 2 months. You are worried about losing your job. You have been prone to headaches since you were a teenager. During that period, you occasionally suffered severe headaches, usually on the left side of your head and often associated with flashing lights. You were told by various doctors that this is migraine but they only occurred occasionally with a tendency for the attacks to coincide at the same time as your periods.

Past medical and surgical history
Nine months ago you were involved in a road traffic accident. You were a passenger in a car which was stationary when another car ran into the back. You developed a sore neck soon after the accident and you have been discussing the possibility of litigation with your lawyer. You wonder if your recent headaches could be related to the accident. Several months after the road traffic accident, your headaches became more severe. They began occurring every day and tend to be felt at the back of your head and radiate round like a tight band. They tend to be better at the weekends but worse during the week. They are throbbing in character and co-codamol and paracetamol tablets are only partly effective.

Other complaints
Menorrhagia (heavy and prolonged periods at regular intervals) for which you have been referred to a gynaecologist.

Current medications
You take up to eight paracetamol and codeine tablets every day.

Relevant previous medications
None.

Social History
You are happily married with two children aged 9 and 13. Both the children are well. You smoke 20 cigarettes per day. Your alcohol consumption is minimal; you drink 2-3 glasses of wine per month. You have never used recreational drugs. You drink four or five cups of coffee a day – this has increased recently because of your stress at work.

Occupational history
Both you and your husband work and you have found your own job increasingly stressful of late. The office has not replaced one of the other secretaries and the extra workload appears to be landing on your shoulders.

Family history
Your father is well but your mother was diagnosed with lung cancer about 2 months ago and has just completed a course of radiotherapy.

Patient's concerns, expectations and wishes
You wish to be reassured that these headaches are not serious and that they can be treated.

| **Lifestyle** |
| You are happily married with two children aged 9 and 13. Both the children are well. You smoke 20 cigarettes per day. Your alcohol consumption is minimal; you drink 2-3 glasses of wine per month. You have never used recreational drugs. You drink four or five cups of coffee a day – this has increased recently because of your stress at work. |
| **Occupational history** |
| Both you and your husband work and you have found your own job increasingly stressful of late. The office has not replaced one of the other secretaries and the extra workload appears to be landing on your shoulders. |
| **Family history** |
| Your father is well but your mother was diagnosed with lung cancer about 2 months ago and has just completed a course of radiotherapy. |
| **Patient's concerns, expectations and wishes** |
| You wish to be reassured that these headaches are not serious and that they can be treated. |
| **You have some specific questions for the doctor at this consultation:** |
| What is causing my headaches?
Could they be due to a brain tumour?
Could they be related to the car accident?
What investigations will I need? |

3.13.3: Examiner Information

| **Probable diagnosis:** |
| Probable chronic persistent ('tension') headache |
| **Plausible alternative diagnosis:** |
| Analgesic induced headache |
| **Key issues to address:** |
| Work stress and family health issues in mother as contributing factors
Consider the role of potential litigation in the presentation
Propose a reasonable management plan which may include brain imaging
Consider the risks of over investigation |

3.14 Case 14

3.14.1   Candidate information

Dear Doctor

Re: Victoria Smythe

Thank you for seeing this 64-year-old librarian who gives a vague history of joint stiffness. She feels tired all the time and has recently developed vague aches and pains. I did prescribe her an anti-depressant although it has not helped her symptoms. I would be grateful for any guidance on her further management.

Yours sincerely

Dr Loomba

You have 14 minutes with the patient and 1 minute for reflection before discussion with the examiners.

Take as detailed a general medical history as possible with emphasis on the cause for complaint

You are not expected to examine the patient.

Case 14

3.14.2   Subject information

You are a 68-year-old retired schoolteacher. You have always been very active and have enjoyed playing tennis. In the last year you have noticed a dramatic deterioration in your health. It started with a flu bug which you had last Christmas and since then you have found it very difficult getting out of bed in the morning. You feel that your body is just as stiff as a board and it can take up to an hour to get out of bed. You seem to have lost your appetite and you have lost over a stone in weight. You feel generally miserable and have confided in your boss that you might be losing your mind.

Your GP gave you anti-depressant drugs although they made you feel drowsy and shaky so you stopped them. They did not make any difference to your symptoms however. In the last two months you have had headaches and find that you can no longer tolerate the hair slides that you have worn for many years as your head seems to have become tender.

Case 14

3.14.3 Examiner information

A key clue in the GP's letter is stiffness and the candidate needs to investigate this thoroughly during the history-taking period. A good candidate would ascertain that the patient actually does have joint stiffness, focusing as to whether this is early morning stiffness or whether the stiffness occurred later on in the day. The GP has been vague in her symptoms although the candidate would need to establish exactly the type of discomfort the patient is experiencing, focusing on co-existing weakness of muscles.

The candidate should ask specifically about any problems with girdle muscles and also muscles of the cervical or lumbar spine. It has to be remembered that hands and feet are never affected in polymyalgia rheumatica. Many patients will complain of symptoms of anorexia and weight loss and also a low-grade fever. Restriction of movement of shoulders and hips is characteristic. The distribution of muscle involvement is bilateral and symmetrical. Occasionally there may be limb muscle involvement. The recent history of headache is very important and it is imperative the candidate works to look for other features of giant cell arteritis. This condition is clinically associated by headaches and temporal tenderness. Early diagnosis and treatment is imperative to prevent blindness.

In terms of investigations there is no specific test for polymyalgia rheumatica. This condition is often a diagnosis of exclusion. This lady would have baseline bloods consisting of an ESR, which is often very high. The ESR is a good tool for effectiveness of treatment as it will return to normal once treatment is initiated. There may be a mild normochromic normocytic anaemia and tests for rheumatoid factor are negative although false positives can be found, especially in elderly people. Giant cell arteritis can occur in up to 40% of patients with polymyalgia rheumatica. Temporal artery biopsy should be requested if this is suspected.

4 Communication Skills & Ethics

Advice to the candidate
This part of the examination may cause you the most anxiety.
Unlike the case histories, which you will be well practised upon simply by your duties as a doctor, the ethics stations can provide you with a multitude of situations which you yourself may never have experienced in this stage of your career

How can you prepare for this?
Learn the ethical ways of thinking
Be prepared for ethical and moral reasoning
Have some idea of certain disease states, occupations and the law
You will not need to have in-depth legal knowledge, but should know of conditions where you may need to notify a disease, or inform the DVLA

All of these areas have been covered in the booklet.
If your practice shows that your main concern is the welfare of the patient which in many of the exam scenario's will need to be balanced against the welfare of the public, you will pass by showing that your advice is based upon ethical reasoning and moral values. You should be aware patient confidentiality and areas where you would be allowed to disclose information to prevent harm.

What are the examiners looking for?
- Someone who is pleasant (in some scenario's, the subject will be asked to become angry and even aggressive). Fear not, no one has been asked to punch you, so stay calm, remain focussed and show that you can empathise with the situation that is causing the subject to behave in this way.
- Many of the subjects in the exam will be specialist nurses, GP's or even research scientists who have some insight to the medical profession
- Be frank with the patient (honesty means integrity), the examiners hate liars!
- When breaking bad news, allow verbal and non-verbal gestures from the subject to change your sensitivity, but not your credibility in being an honest doctor
- When presenting to the examiner, you must show that you are willing to seek advice from authorities for difficult situations. After all in reality you would not and should not be left to deal with some ethical dilemmas and your consultant would carry the can for this. You must still show that you are able to communicate and do all the groundwork in ascertaining
    - What the subject wants
    - What the subject needs
    - What can be done?
    - What should be done?
    - What are you going to do
- For most scenario's you should have reached a plan at the closure of the interview. This does not always mean a conclusion. A realistic feasible plan will be what is sort after in many of these scenarios.
- On studying the scenarios, you will be given insight of what the subject has been told, and also what the examiner is looking for and you should practice thinking ethically as well as clinically.
- All GMC based dilemmas and many Royal college type scenarios have been covered

4.1 Case 1

Problem: Driving when medically unfit

4.1.1 Candidate Information

Role: You are the medical SHO on-call and asked by the A&E staff to attend a patient who has presented a hypoglycaemic attack.
Please read the scenario below. You may make notes on the paper provided. When the bell sounds, enter the examination room.

Subject definition: Mr Watkins is an HGV driver who is taking insulin.

Scenario
He has had some intravenous dextrose, and is now awake and oriented. This is the first hypoglycaemic episode which has required hospital treatment.

Your task is to convince Mr Watkins of the need to revoke his driving licence and persuade him to inform the DVLA.

Instructions to Candidate
- You have 14 minutes until the patient/subject leaves the room followed by 1 minute for reflection before discussion with the examiners.
- Do <u>not</u> take the history again except for details that will help in your discussion with the patient.
- *You are not required to examine the patient/subject.*

Case 1

4.1.2 Subject Information

Role: You are Mr Lesley Watkins

Subject Definition: You work for a small local company where you have been employed for 10 years as an HGV driver, making deliveries throughout the United Kingdom. You are 50 years old. Prior to taking this job, you were unemployed for 12 years following a redundancy at a company you joined shortly after leaving school. You have no other formal qualifications or skills.

This job has saved you from financial ruin.

You are married and have 4 school aged children who live at home.

You are the main earner in the family and pay a mortgage. Your wife works part time because she takes the children to and from school.

Your salary enables you to live comfortably and you enjoy your working environment

Scenario:
One year ago, you developed an illness, which left you exhausted. You collapsed and were taken to hospital where you were told that you had diabetes. You were told you would have to take insulin for the rest of your life. The nurse specialist explained that you would need to notify the driving authorities and that it is likely that you would lose your HGV licence, and thus you would have to change your job. You decided to ignore this advice as unemployment in the area is high and you are not trained for any other role.

All had gone well until the past week and you had controlled your diabetes meticulously .However, on the day in question you had been out playing football with the children and were late taking lunch. As a result you had collapsed and an ambulance had been called to take you to the A&E Department where you were treated for hypoglycaemia. You realise the cause of the hypoglycaemia and had always been scrupulously careful to avoid such a problem while working.

When the doctor suggests you need to inform the authorities, you refuse point blank. You become irritated but not aggressive. Try to negotiate the doctor around to colluding with you, and not mentioning this to the authorities or your employers.

Case 1

4.1.3 Examiner Information

Problem: Driving When Medically Unfit
If the candidate appears to have finished early, remind them how long is left at the station and enquire if there is anything else they would like to ask, or whether they have finished.   If they have finished, please allow the candidate that time for reflection and remain silent. The patient should remain until the end of the 14-minute period.

A good candidate would be expected to have agreed a summary and plan of action with the subject before closure.   Nonetheless, in discussion, the examiners will usually ask the candidate (after 1 minute's reflection) to summarise the problems raised in the foregoing exchange.

The candidate should be expected to:
* Explain the situation clearly and in a non-patronising manner, without using jargon.
* Clearly explain the problems of continuing to drive whilst recognising the patient's dilemma.
* Explain that it is not legal to maintain an HGV licence whilst on insulin.
* Advise the patient to inform the licensing authorities.
* Remain calm in the face of mild aggressive and emotional behaviour by the patient.
* Agree a plan by the end of the interview.
* Begin to explore other career options.

The candidate should be asked to identify the ethical and/or legal issues raised in this case and how they would address them. The framework for discussion should include consideration of the four underlying ethical principles.
* Respect of the patient's autonomy (ie the capacity of the patient to make deliberated or reasoned decisions for himself and to act on the basis of those decisions)
* Disclosure of confidential information. In this situation, it is in the best interest of the public if this information is handed to the relevant authorities. The doctor would not need the patients consent in this situation.
* Beneficence: Duty to do good and a moral obligation to do no harm
* Duty to act justly
* Legal aspects – a detailed knowledge of medical law is *not* required.

The candidate should recognise their limit in dealing with problem and know when, and from where, to seek further advice and support.

Candidates must demonstrate competent performance in all domains outlined in the marking schedule in order to pass this station.

4.1.4 Tutorial: Driving & Diabetes
(The information has been reproduced from Diabetes UK booklet "Driving & Diabetes" - 1997.)

Having diabetes does not mean that you need to give up driving. But it does mean that you need to plan in advance before you get behind the wheel.

Informing the DVLA : Advice for patient.
If you have diabetes which is treated with insulin or tablets, you must, by law, inform the Driver and Vehicle Licensing Agency (DVLA) soon after you have been diagnosed. You must also inform them if you have had diabetes for some time and are applying for a licence, perhaps for the first time. And you must inform them if any problems or diabetic complications develop which may affect your ability to drive.

If your diabetes is treated by diet alone, you do not need to inform them, but you must inform them if your treatment changes - for example, from diet alone to diet and tablets.

When you apply for a licence, the application form will ask whether you have, or have ever had, any of a number of medical problems. Answer YES to the questions asking about diabetes. When asked to give details, say whether your diabetes is treated by tablets, and or insulin.

After you have filled in and returned your application form, you will be sent another form (called 'Diabetic I') asking for more information and for the name and address of your GP and/or hospital doctor. You will also be asked to fill in a consent form so that the DVLA can approach your doctor directly if necessary. People who treat their diabetes with tablets are not always sent this form.

This procedure does not mean that you will be refused a driving licence. The DVLA just needs to be sure that every licensed driver is going to be safe on the road. So as long as your diabetes is well controlled, and you have no complications which might impair your safety as a driver - and your doctor confirms this if asked - there is no reason why you should not be issued with a licence. It is important that you answer the questions honestly.

If you have a motorcycle, the rules for informing the DVLA are the same as those for a car.

Restricted licences
If you take insulin you will be issued with a licence for one, two or three years. Just before the expiry date, you will receive a reminder to renew and you will be asked to return your current licence. You may also be sent another 'Diabetic I' form (see above) to confirm your medical condition. Renewals of restricted licences are supplied free of charge.

If you are treated with tablets or diet alone, you will be issued with an 'until 70' licence (unless any other medical conditions rule this out). When this licence expires, you will need to renew it every one to three years, just like other people in the UK who are over 70 years old.

Insurance cover
You must tell your insurers that you have diabetes - whether or not there is a question on the proposal form specifically about diabetes or not.
Failure to do so can invalidate your cover in the event of a claim.

Not all insurers will offer insurance cover to people with diabetes. Of those that do, some may impose special terms or charge an increased premium. If this happens, it is worth challenging your insurer, especially if your diabetes is stable and well controlled.

Do not drive you have just started to take insulin and your diabetes is not yet properly controlled. Your doctor or diabetes specialist nurse will be able to give you more advice on this.

Also:
➢ If you have difficulty in recognising the early symptoms of hypoglycaemia.
➢ If you have any problems with your eyesight that cannot be corrected by glasses.
➢ If you have numbness or weakness in your limbs caused by neuropathy

You should avoid long or stressful journeys if you are tired.

Hypoglycaemia (low blood glucose)
There is a risk of hypoglycaemia if your diabetes is treated with insulin or with sulphonylurea tablets (such as Glibenclamide, Gliclazide, Chlorpropamide or Glipizide). Having a hypo while you are in charge of a motor vehicle can be fatal, not only for you, but for others as well. Whether driving or not, you should always carry some form of glucose with you in your pocket or handbag. Keep glucose tablets plus biscuits, fruit or sandwiches in the car.

You can avoid hypoglycaemia by:
➢ Never driving for more than two hours without stopping for a snack.
➢ Not delaying or missing a meal or snack.
➢ Checking your blood glucose before and during a journey.

If you feel hypoglycaemic
The symptoms of hypoglycaemia may include hunger, sweating, shakiness, palpitations, faintness, dizziness, nausea or a headache. Sometimes you may notice double vision or tingling around the lips.

At the first signs of hypoglycaemia:
➢ STOP driving as soon as it is safe to do so. Do not attempt to start again until the symptoms have disappeared.
➢ Take glucose tablets, biscuits or some other form of carbohydrate immediately.
➢ Make it clear that you are no longer in charge of the car by leaving the driving seat, stepping out of the car (if safe to do so) and by removing the ignition key. This is to refute any suggestion that you are in charge of a car whilst under the influence of any drugs including insulin.

If you have an accident
If you do have a hypoglycaemic episode at the wheel, you may be charged with driving under the influence of a drug, insulin, driving without due care and attention, or dangerous driving. Therefore, it is essential that you check your blood glucose levels to make sure this does not happen. If you are prosecuted, we recommend that you seek legal advice immediately.

Whatever the outcome, the DVLA may revoke your driving licence. The driver has the right to appeal to the court to have the licence restored, but in order to succeed the court must be convinced that the incident was due to most unusual circumstances and that the onset of another uncontrolled hypoglycaemic episode whilst driving is unlikely. A doctor's report to this effect can be most helpful so it is important to discuss the circumstances with your doctor if you have an accident due to hypoglycaemia.

<u>Driving large goods vehicles and passenger carrying vehicles</u>
People whose diabetes is treated by diet alone or diet and tablets are normally allowed to hold LGV and PCV licences, provided they are otherwise in good health. (Until 1991 these were known as heavy goods vehicles [HGV] and public service vehicles [PSV1).

People treated with insulin are not allowed to have these licences. If you currently hold such a licence and start using insulin, you must inform the DVLA and stop driving the vehicle immediately.

The only exception is if you had IDDM and were issued with such a licence before April 1991 when the law changed. If you were, and are now refused renewal, you can appeal to the DVLA and, if this is unsuccessful, you can take the matter to the Magistrates Court. The DVLA will explain the appeal procedure to you.

4.2   Case 2

Problem: **Disclosure of information**

4.2.1 Candidate Information

Role: You are the medical SHO on-call in A&E. You are asked to see a frequent attendee who has come in with excruciating abdominal pain. This man is a known heroin addict and has been seen by the surgeons who are happy to discharge him. He does have an area of cellulitis, which they believe the medics can treat.

As you assess him, he tries to convince you that he is having opiate withdrawal and has lost his methadone. You are satisfied that his condition is stable. You complete your review and leave him for a few moments to write in the notes and he absconds.

Please read the scenario below. You may make notes on the paper provided. When the bell sounds, enter the examination room.

Subject definition: Disclosure of information to the law

Scenario
This man is now in police custody for with-holding information about his identity. He has committed a minor traffic offence. His description is unquestionable as he is the only man in Tooting with a spider web tattooed on his head.   The police Officer has come to discuss his identity with you.

Instructions to Candidate
- You have 14 minutes until the patient/subject leaves the room followed by 1 minute for reflection before discussion with the examiners.
- Do <u>not</u> take the history again except for details that will help in your discussion with the patient.
- *You are not required to examine the patient/subject.*

Case 2

4.2.2 Subject Information

Role: You are Chief Inspector Booth

You are the Sergeant on duty at Tooting Police Station.

Subject Definition: Disclosure of confidential information

Scenario:
2 hours ago, you received a 999 call from a local residence to report an attempted robbery.

On arrival at the scene, the culprit had absconded but fortunately, nothing was taken and no one was hurt.

On leaving the premises, you observed someone behaving suspiciously in what appeared to be a stolen car.

On following him, he committed a minor road traffic offence and was cautioned.
At this time, he was found to have several mobile phones, jewellery in his car boot.
He claimed that the items were his own but refused to give any other information.
He was arrested and currently in custody at the police station.

He informed the staff at the police station that he was unwell and had just been discharged from hospital.

The Medical cover doctor at the police station was satisfied that there was nothing wrong with him.

He had refused to give any other information, but there were suspicions that he had been mugging and robbing innocent people to maintain his drug habit.

This man fits the description of a menace, who you believe is wanted for a number of charges of minor thefts.

You are eager to arrest this man for theft and robbery and would like to know more about him from casualty staff.

You try to convince them of what a danger he is.

Case 2

4.2.3 Examiner Information

Subject: Disclosure of information without consent

If the candidate appears to have finished early, remind them how long is left at the station and enquire if there is anything else they would like to ask, or whether they have finished. If they have finished, please allow the candidate that time for reflection and remain silent. The patient should remain until the end of the 14-minute period.

A good candidate would
- Communicate professionally with the police constable
- The doctor should explain that the hospital admission itself is not suspicious malicious criminal behaviour, and that any other information about the patient is confidential.
- In the view of the road traffic offence, the doctor Must breach confidentiality and provide the police constable with the name and address of the patient (Road traffic act 1988)
- This does not include clinical details and in informing the police of these, the doctor would have breached confidentiality, which is not legally acceptable.
- The doctor must explain that, he cannot without the patients consent divulge any other information which could be used to prevent minor crime, or to help conviction in minor crime. Most crimes against properties are considered to be minor crimes now.
- Similarly the doctor cannot breach confidentiality to prevent minor harm to another individual.

The candidate should be asked to identify the ethical and/or legal issues raised in this case and how they would address them. The framework for discussion should include consideration of the four underlying ethical principles.
- Respect of the patient's autonomy (ie the capacity of the patient to make deliberated or reasoned decisions for himself and to act on the basis of those decisions)
- Disclosure of confidential information. In this situation to divulge any more information,
- the doctor would not need the patients consent in this situation.
- Beneficence: Duty to do good and a moral obligation to do no harm
- Duty to act justly
- Legal aspects – a detailed knowledge of medical law is *not* required.

The candidate should recognise their limit in dealing with problem and know when, and from where, to seek further advice and support.

Candidates must demonstrate competent performance in all domains outlined in the marking schedule in order to pass this station.

4.3 Case 3

Problem: **Resuscitation Decision**

4.3.1 Candidate Information

Role: You are the medical SHO doing a ward round. You have been told by the nurses that the wife of one of your patients would like to speak to you before you review her husband.

He has severe Chronic Obstructive Pulmonary Disease and has been admitted with an infective exacerbation.

He is on home nebulisers, home oxygen and is house bound due to a combination of his lung disease and depression.

On the ward, he is receiving intravenous antibiotics and an aminophyline infusion as well as his nebs and oxygen.

Please read the scenario below. You may make notes on the paper provided. When the bell sounds, enter the examination room.

Subject definition: Mrs Smith does not want her husband to be resuscitated in the event of a cardiac arrest.

Scenario

Mrs Smith is depressed, tired and fed up with her husband's illness. She feels that whilst she would like to continue to care for him, she also can't watch him suffer anymore.

She would like to discuss his resuscitation status with you but does not want him to know, as it would upset him.

She feels that he should not be resuscitated but would like this decision to be made without her husband.

Your task is to explain that whilst resuscitation is likely to be futile, Mr Smith must be involved in all decisions regarding his care and that will include discussions about his resuscitation.

Instructions to Candidate
- You have 14 minutes until the patient/subject leaves the room followed by 1 minute for reflection before discussion with the examiners.
- Do <u>not</u> take the history again except for details that will help in your discussion with the patient.
- *You are not required to examine the patient/subject.*

Case 3

4.3.2 Subject Information

Role: You are Mrs Smith

Subject Definition:
You are a 42 year old woman who suffers from angina and arthritis affecting your knees and your back.

Scenario:
Your husband, who is 67, has suffered from lung disease for 40 years.

He smoked from the age of 13 until last year when he finally gave up.

He has been admitted to hospital over 20 times in the last 3 years and has a very poor quality of life.

He is on home nebulisers and oxygen.

You are the main carer for your husband and you have chosen this role for yourself.

You do however find it exhausting.

You have not had a holiday for 3 years because your husband refuses respite care. He is house bound and can only just manage to dress himself and mobilise a little in the house.

Your only outings together these days are in the ambulance when he is brought to casualty.

You are afraid to go out for more than an hour at a time because he panics and his breathing gets bad.

You hate to see him this way and know that he will not live long.

You would like him to die naturally and don't want doctors to prolong his life only to increase his suffering.

You want the doctors to decide not to resuscitate him but don't want him to be involved in the decision making.

Case 3
4.3.3 Examiner Information

Problem: Making a DNR decision
If the candidate appears to have finished early, remind them how long is left at the station and enquire if there is anything else they would like to ask, or whether they have finished.   If they have finished, please allow the candidate that time for reflection and remain silent. The patient should remain until the end of the 14-minute period.

A good candidate would be expected to have agreed a summary and plan of action with the subject before closure.   Nonetheless, in discussion, the examiners will usually ask the candidate (after 1 minute's reflection) to summarise the problems raised in the foregoing exchange.

The candidate should be expected to:
- Explore Mr Smith's previous history including his quality of life
- Explain the current medical situation
- Recognising the subjects dilemma
- Explain that resuscitation attempts are likely to be futile
- Stress that Mr Smith must be fully informed of any discussions about his care and that includes decisions made regarding resuscitation
- Suggest that her husband may also have concerns and that they should try to discuss it together

The candidate should be asked to identify the ethical and/or legal issues raised in this case and how they would address them. The framework for discussion should include consideration of the four underlying ethical principles.
- Respect of the patient's autonomy (i.e. the capacity of the patient to make deliberated or reasoned decisions for himself and to act on the basis of those decisions)
- Disclosure of confidential information. In this situation, the doctor does not need the patients consent to discuss his illness with his wife and carer.
- Beneficence: Duty to do good and a moral obligation to do no harm. Not providing CPR would be equivalent to withdrawing life prolonging treatment.
- Duty to act justly
- Legal aspects – a detailed knowledge of medical law is *not* required.

The candidate should recognise their limit in dealing with problem and know when, and from where, to seek further advice and support.

Candidates must demonstrate competent performance in all domains outlined in the marking schedule in order to pass this station.

4.4 Case 4

Problem: **Discussing a Post Mortem**

4.4.1 Candidate Information

Role: You are Care of the Elderly SHO. You have been looking after Mr Gibbs, an 42 year old gentleman who died unexpectedly from a cardiac arrest last night. You were not on call and can only ascertain from the notes that this was an asystolic arrest which was managed appropriately by the on call crash team. He had been undergoing investigations as an inpatient for severe back pain, which was thought to be due to metastatic disease. The primary had not been found. He was due to have a CT of his abdomen this week

Please read the scenario below. You may make notes on the paper provided. When the bell sounds, enter the examination room.

Subject definition: Breaking bad news and requesting post mortem

Scenario

His wife has come to the ward to speak with you after his death.

She has not spoken to any doctor yet but received a call from the nursing staff in the early hours of the morning. A neighbour kindly brought her to hospital when she was informed of the death.

Your Consultant would be interested to know the cause of his symptoms and has asked you to request a Post Mortem examination.

Instructions to Candidate
- You have 14 minutes until the patient/subject leaves the room followed by 1 minute for reflection before discussion with the examiners.
- Do not take the history again except for details that will help in your discussion with the patient.
- *You are not required to examine the patient/subject.*

Case 4

4.4.2 Subject Information

Role: You are Mrs Gibbs

Subject Definition:
You are 40 years old and work as a Headmistress at a local private school.

Scenario:

You and your husband have always enjoyed good health.

Your husband developed excruciating back pain one month ago while on a sailing holiday. Initially it was thought that he had pulled a muscle but as it got worse, the GP requested an X Ray of his back.

There was some concern that this may be bone cancer and he was referred to the outpatients' clinic last week. He was admitted from clinic to have further tests.

He had a number of tests, which were all inconclusive, but there was a mention on discussion with the consultant that he may have cancer that had spread to his bones. During his life, your husband had never complained of any other symptoms. He had always enjoyed his food; he played squash every week and had a very good job as a bank manager.

He had felt a little under the weather on holiday but it was not in his nature to make a fuss.

The thought of him having cancer had worried you both after the Consultant ward round but you were hoping that the tests he was to have would have come back clear.

You were phoned by the sister on the ward at 5 am asking you to come to hospital.

On arrival you were told that your husband had died. His heart had stopped beating.

The doctor suggests a post mortem examination.

You are not sure exactly what this is or why the hospital need to do it.

You are not so sure that you want to know any more about the cause of death.

You need an explanation of what the examination is and how it will be of benefit to anyone if at all.

You have heard that coroners are people that ask for post-mortems and would like to know if a coroner has been involved.

Case 4

4.4.3 Examiner Information

Problem: Breaking bad news and requesting a post mortem

If the candidate appears to have finished early, remind them how long is left at the station and enquire if there is anything else they would like to ask, or whether they have finished.   If they have finished, please allow the candidate that time for reflection and remain silent. The patient should remain until the end of the 14-minute period. A good candidate would be expected to have agreed a summary and plan of action with the subject before closure. Nonetheless, in discussion, the examiners will usually ask the candidate (after 1 minute's reflection) to summarise the problems raised in the foregoing exchange. The candidate should be expected to:

- Express condolence and appreciate that the subject has sustained a major loss
- Ascertain how much emotional support the subject has in dealing with this bereavement
- Allow the subject to speak and ask questions which should by answered with sensitivity and empathy
- Explain the cause of death which was a cardiac arrest. This may or may not have been related to the symptoms that were being investigated. Explain what happens at an arrest and reassure that all active measures were taken to prevent death
- Express doubt as to the insight of the underlying disease
- Explain what a post mortem involves and what information it may yield
- Allow for her not to make an informed and non-pressurised decision and also to discuss this with relatives before making a final decision

The candidate should be asked to identify the ethical and/or legal issues raised in this case and how they would address them. The framework for discussion should include consideration of the following underlying ethical considerations.

- In order to give consent to such a procedure, the subject must competent and show capacity to agree to examination
- The subject must be given all relevant information
- Beneficence: Duty to do good and a moral obligation to do no harm. Be prepared to be honest that a postmortem of this nature would be mainly of an academic interest which may prove useful in the diagnosis of future patients
- Duty to act justly
- Legal aspects – a detailed knowledge of medical law is *not* required.

The candidate should recognise their limit in dealing with problem and know when, and from where, to seek further advice and support.
Candidates must demonstrate competent performance in all domains outlined in the marking schedule in order to pass this station.

What is a Post-mortem?

In certain situations when someone dies, it may be necessary to carry out a post-mortem examination (also called an autopsy) of the deceased's body. A post-mortem examination is a medical examination of a dead body to determine the exact cause of death.

Such examinations are only requested if:
- There has been a serious uncertainty about the cause of death.
- Examination will provide vital answers as to the cause of death.

In the case of a violent death, the post-mortem may be necessary as part of a criminal investigation. Post-mortems are carried out by a specific type of Physician called a 'pathologist'.

It's important to remember that during a post-mortem examination, the body is treated with utmost respect and no disfigurement of the body takes place. In fact, the body may be viewed afterwards, and usually should not delay funeral arrangements.

The family or next of kin will normally be asked for their permission before a post-mortem is carried out. However, where a Coroner has ordered a post-mortem examination, the permission of the next of kin is not necessary.

Coroners will request post-mortem examinations in instances where the death is suspicious, sudden and unexpected or unexplainable.

During a post-mortem examination, all body cavities (head, chest and abdomen) are examined and the organs dissected. Small blocks of tissue and blood samples may be retained by the pathologist for further examination. Occasionally, it may be necessary for the pathologist to retain a whole organ (or organs) for more detailed examination in order to establish the cause of death. Where an organ is retained, this is purely for the purpose of establishing or clearly determining the cause of death. Consent of the next-of-kin is not required, but they will be notified. In addition, the next-of-kin will be required to express a preference for ultimate disposal of any organs removed. Retention of an organ for any other purposes by a pathologist (i.e., teaching, research, etc.) requires specific consent from the next-of kin.

Following the postmortem examination, the body will normally be released to the spouse or next-or-kin immediately after the examination has been completed

Although the need for a postmortem will not usually delay the funeral, the results may not be available until three to eight weeks later. In certain circumstances, it may be several weeks before the postmortem report is received from the pathologist. For example, in situations where a toxicology (drug) screen is required it may be several months before the postmortem report is completed. Queries relating to postmortem reports should be made to the Coroner's office and not to the hospital concerned.

You can discuss the results with the deceased's doctor once the results are available, and you can then proceed with registering the death in the usual way. You cannot register the death until the postmortem results are received by the Coroner's Office. Prior to inquest (or whilst awaiting the postmortem report) the Coroner will provide on request an Interim Certificate of the Fact of Death. (This may be acceptable to banks, insurance companies and other institutions but you should check with the institutions for their requirements).

4.5 Case 5

Problem: Breaking the news to a patient who has multiple sclerosis.

4.5.1 Candidate Information

Role: You are the general medicine SHO on duty that assists the visiting neurologist at his weekly clinic. In the neurologist's absence, you have been called to the Outpatients Department.

Please read the scenario below. You may make notes on the paper provided. When the bell sounds, enter the examination room.
Subject definition: Patient who is about to be told they have multiple sclerosis.
Scenario:

Miss Susan Hinds, a 35 year old Practice nurse has been referred by her GP with a history of recurrent visual disturbance, transient weakness, tiredness and lethargy. On examination, she has an internuclear ophthalmoplegia. Investigations showing oligoclonal bands in the CSF and MRI scan showing demyelination indicate a diagnosis of multiple sclerosis have recently been undertaken. She has come back to the clinic before the day of her appointment, as she is concerned to know the results of her tests.

Your task is to break this news to Miss Hinds
- You have 14 minutes until the patient/subject leaves the room followed by 1 minute for reflection before discussion with the examiners.
- Do <u>not</u> take the history again except for details that will help in your discussion with the patient.
- *You are not required to examine the patient/subject.*

Case 5

4.5.2 Subject Information

Role: You are a patient about to be told you have multiple sclerosis.
Scenario:

You are Susan Hinds, a 35 year old nurse for a local General Practitioner. You have been suffering from transient symptoms of blurred vision, tiredness and lethargy.
In the first instance you thought that you were over working and took a few days off work.

This was a year ago and the symptoms have recurred several times, lasting days and sometimes weeks.

You went to the opticians to get better glasses for fear that this was all due to eye strain but even after spending a fortune, the blurry vision has recurred.

You have had periods of time with no symptoms. However, recently you had a bout, which kept you off work for 2 weeks and went to your GP. You were referred to the Neurology Department and had a series of investigation including a lumbar puncture and a MRI scan. You have come to the Outpatients Department today for the results, as you are concerned. Your appointment is for next week and you do not realise that the consultant neurologist is not here every day.

Prior to this, you have always been well.

You are on the contraceptive pill, and no other regular medication. You are planning to marry your long term boyfriend and start a family within a year or two.

You believe your problems are due to a combination of stress and maybe 'viral' as you come into contact with so many patients.

You have become concerned by all elaborate tests and although you have heard about multiple sclerosis, it has never entered your mind that you may be suffering from something quite so serious. Your main concern is to get well so that you can house-hunt and become pregnant.

You are stunned to hear what the doctor says and deeply upset.

Initially you are in denial and ask him if he has the correct case notes.

You can't take on board what he is saying and frequently have to ask him to repeat what he has just said.

You are worried as to how you will break this news to your partner and parents.

You want to know if it will affect your chances to have a baby.

Case 5

4.5.3 Examiner Information

Problem: Patient that is about to be told they have multiple sclerosis.
If the candidate appears to have finished early, remind them how long is left at the station and enquire if there is anything else they would like to ask, or whether they have finished.   If they have finished, please allow the candidate that time for reflection and remain silent. The patient should remain silent until the end of the 14-minute period.

A good candidate would be expected to have agreed a summary and plan of action with the subject before closure.   Nonetheless, in discussion, the examiners will usually ask the candidate (after 1 minute's reflection) to summarise the problems raised in the foregoing exchange.

The candidates should be able to explain the diagnosis of M.S. and its likely consequences in a sympathetic and empathetic manner. The candidate should be able to explain the uncertain prognosis of M.S., and the treatment options currently available – this should include the issues of pregnancy and potential disability. The candidate should conduct the interview recognising the verbal and non-verbal cues of anxiety and distress shown by the patient.

The candidate would be expected to explain, whether prompted or not, some of the long term implications, striking an appropriate balance between realism and optimism; the importance of a support network of family, friends and agencies now and in the future. The candidate should be asked to identify the ethical and/or legal issues raised in this case and how they would address them. The framework for discussion should include consideration of the four underlying ethical principles:
- Respect of the patient's autonomy
- Duty to do good and not to do harm
- Duty to act justly
- Legal aspects – a detailed knowledge of medical law is *not* required.

The candidate should recognise their limit in dealing with a problem and know when, and from where, to seek further advice and support.

Candidates must demonstrate competent performance in all domains outlined in the marking schedule in order to pass this station.

4.6 Case 6

Problem: Male patient with symptoms suggestive of colonic carcinoma.

4.6.1 Candidate Information

Role: You are the SHO in a busy outpatient clinic. You are about to see Mr Bland who presented with the following GP letter:

"Thank you for seeing Mr Bland so promptly. He is a 54 year old Accountant who I have seen after many years. He came to see me yesterday having noticed some rectal bleeding for the past month. This has been associated with an altered bowel habit and I am concerned that he may have cancer."

Please read the scenario below (you may make notes if you wish on the paper provided).   When the bell sounds, enter the examination room to begin the consultation.

Subject definition: Male patient with symptoms suggestive of colonic carcinoma

Scenario:
You have seen Mr Bland who presented with the following symptoms:
- Lethargy, dizziness and fatigue
- Anorexia
- Weight loss
- Altered bowel habit with a tendency towards constipation and occasional diarrhoea
- Rectal bleeding

Whilst these symptoms should alert you to investigate the patient in order to diagnose or exclude carcinoma, you cannot imply the diagnosis without further tests.

You are asked to confirm the story and then decide what to say to the patient at this stage. Mr Bland is eager to know what is going on.

- You have 14 minutes until the patient/subject leaves the room followed by 1 minute for reflection before discussion with the examiners.
- Do not take the history again except for details that will help in your discussion with the patient.
- *You are not required to examine the patient/subject.*

Case 6

4.6.2 Subject Information

Role: You are Mr Bland. You have been sent urgently to the outpatient clinic by your GP because of a problem with your bowels.

Subject definition: Patient Mr Bland

You are 54 year old accountant who has recently remarried. You have 2 children from your first marriage, who are both away at university. Your wife died from breast cancer 9 years ago. You have married a colleague who is 36. You met at your church and became close after she became a widow 5 years ago. She has 2 children aged 6 and 7 whom you love as your own.

You smoke the occasional cigar.

Scenario

Your concern is that for the past month weeks you have felt worn out and are exhausted without doing anything. You feel dizzy and have lost your appetite. You have now noticed periods of constipation and loose bowel action, sometimes with blood mixed in with the stool.

You want to know what is going on. You want to know if it is serious, particularly as you are the main provider for your wife and children.

Case 6

4.6.3 Examiner Information

Problem: male patient with symptoms suggestive of colonic cancer.

If the candidate appears to have finished early, remind them how long is left at the station and enquire if there is anything else they would like to ask, or whether they have finished.   If they have finished, please allow the candidate that time for reflection and remain silent. The patient should remain until the end of the 14-minute period.

A good candidate would be expected to have agreed a summary and plan of action with the subject before closure.   Nonetheless, in discussion, the examiners will usually ask the candidate (after 1 minute's reflection) to summarise the problems raised in the foregoing exchange.

In the past it would have been argued that the best interests of the patient would not be served by sharing with him, at this stage, the possibility of cancer. This could lead to problems in the doctor/patient relationship later.

A good candidate will be open, straightforward, and share information to develop a co-operative relationship in which Mr Jones will be prepared for a later discussion concerning diagnosis and treatment options. The doctor in this case could say, "I'd like to arrange for you to have some tests to find out why you are bleeding. It could be something quite simple, e.g. a polyp, or it could be a more serious problem, in which case we shall want to do something about it as soon as we can."

The candidate should be asked to identify the ethical and/or legal issues raised in this case and how they would address them. The framework for discussion should include consideration of the four underlying ethical principles:
- Respect for the patient's autonomy
- Duty to do good and not to do harm
- Duty to act justly
- Legal aspects – a detailed knowledge of medical law is *not* required.

The candidate should recognise their limit in dealing with a problem and know when, and from where, to seek further advice and support.

Candidates must demonstrate competent performance in all domains outlined in the marking schedule in order to pass this station.

4.7 Case 7

4.7.1 Candidate Information

Role: You are the medical SHO on call. You are asked to come urgently to the A&E Department where Mrs Khan Brown has presented with 24 hours of haemoptysis and a two-month history of cough, purulent sputum and weight loss.

Please read the scenario below. You may make notes on the paper provided. When the bell sounds, enter the examination room.

Subject definition: Patient Mrs Khan aged 40.

Scenario:
Urgent staining of the sputum has revealed plentiful Mycobacteria (Ziehl-Neelson stain). The A&E SHO says that previous notes of the patient had been found and that a diagnosis of rifampicin and isoniazid resistant tuberculosis and been made 18 months previously. The patient had taken treatment for three months in an isolation unit in hospital before going home. She had been lost to follow up and discontinued treatment after discharge.

The patient is not keen to be admitted as she did not enjoy isolation and would prefer to be at home, looking after her disabled husband.

Your task is to discuss with the patient:
- The need for further investigation (including contributory underlying factors)
- The need for treatment
- The need for admission
- What needs to be done for the household contacts?

Instructions to Candidate
- You have 14 minutes until the patient/subject leaves the room followed by 1 minute for reflection before discussion with the examiners.
- Do not take the history again except for details that will help in your discussion with the patient.
- *You are not required to examine the patient/subject.*

Case 7

Examiner Information

Problem: Multiple Drug Resistant TB: The need to treat.

If the candidate appears to have finished early, remind them how long is left at the station and enquire if there is anything else they would like to ask, or whether they have finished.   If they have finished, please allow the candidate that time for reflection and remain silent. The patient should remain until the end of the 14-minute period.

A good candidate would be expected to have agreed a summary and plan of action with the subject before closure.   Nonetheless, in discussion, the examiners will usually ask the candidate (after 1 minute's reflection) to summarise the problems raised in the foregoing exchange.

This scenario is designed to assess communication skills and ethical knowledge **_not_** knowledge of the treatment of MDR TB. The patient has been asked to be anxious and to feel guilty about not completing the treatment as prescribed previously.

The objective is to assess the skills of the candidate at:
- Explaining the situation
- Negotiating a management outcome
- Conceding (if only temporarily) the need to do an HIV test as this is of secondary importance to the immediate need of isolation and treatment of TB
- Knowledge of the patient's right to refuse treatment ordinarily, but in this case there is an issue of public health. (Section 37 of the Public Health Act 1984, magistrates orders to allow compulsory treatment of a patient with notifiable disease.   This is almost never needed if appropriate negotiation with the patient is undertaken, which is a good thing as it is very difficult to work)
- Knowledge of the issues and sensitivities and HIV testing without informed consent.

The candidate should be asked to identify the ethical and/or legal issues raised in this case and how they would address them. The framework for discussion should include consideration of the four underlying ethical principles:
- Respect of the patient's autonomy
- Duty to do good and not to do harm
- Duty to act justly
- Legal aspects – detailed knowledge of medical law is *not* required.

The candidate should recognise their limit in dealing with a problem and know when, and from where, to seek further advice and support.

Candidates must demonstrate competent performance in all domains outlined in the marking schedule in order to pass this station.

Case 7

4.7.2 Subject Information

Role: You are Mrs Khan aged 40. You started to cough blood yesterday and are now in the A&E Department.

Subject Definition
You work for a charity helping recent immigrants settle into your neighbourhood. You live in a flat with two bedrooms with your disabled partner and your two children, aged 6 and 4.

Scenario
Three years ago you were feeling unwell and found to have tuberculosis and after several attempts to treat you the bacterium became resistant to some of the drugs which had been used. You were referred to an isolation unit in the hospital for treatment in a "negative pressure room" and were not allowed out of the room for three months until your phlegm/sputum no longer contained infectious bacteria. The treatment was with six drugs initially (one an injection into your muscle each day) and the tablets made you feel sick. It is not an experience you wish to repeat. After discharge from hospital you went back to your job, which was very stressful, and failed to complete the course of anti-tuberculous therapy which was hard to take (18 pills spaced out in the day) and made you feel unwell.

Two months ago you started to cough again and realised your health was not as good but only admitted to yourself that you were ill again when you started to cough blood yesterday. You are now in the A&E Department and the doctor from the admitting medical team has been asked to come and see you. You are frightened at the prospect of having tuberculosis again but feel guilty that you did not complete the treatment last time. You hope it is not tuberculosis, particularly drug resistant tuberculosis, which will mean you have to be isolated for a long time and take a difficult course of treatment for two years.

You are worried your partner and children may have become infected and want to be reassured they can be seen, assessed and, if necessary, treated as soon as possible. You would like to be with them to help and ask why you cannot be treated at home (like many other people with TB). You know you were HIV negative when you were treated 18 months ago because you agreed to be tested "at the doctor's request". You hope you have remained negative but are anxious since you know you will be asked again and would like to refuse.

Apart from the tuberculosis, you have never been seriously ill. You have never used drugs intravenously for recreational purposes, have not had a blood transfusion and have not travelled extensively outside Europe. You have had unprotected sexual intercourse with another man 9 months ago, and know that this man has had other relationships and has never been tested HIV. You smoke 20 cigarettes a day and are worried you will not be allowed to smoke in hospital. Both children are in school and neighbours and your sister who lives nearby will help your partner to look after them.

N.B. Your main feelings are anxiety and guilt at not completing treatment the first time, *not anger.*

Please agree to the need to admit and treat after appropriate negotiation.

4.8 Case 8

Problem: **Advanced metastatic breast cancer needing referral to oncology services.**

4.8.1 Candidate Information

Role: You are the SHO on the medical ward to which Mrs Hazel, who was admitted 3 days ago. You need to explain to her, that she has advanced metastatic breast cancer, which would be more appropriately treated by the oncologists. You need to explain both the diagnosis and also the reason why you wish to refer her to the oncology services.

Please read the scenario below. You may make notes on the paper provided.

When the bell sounds, enter the examination room.

Subject definition: Mrs Hazel is a 50 year old married English teacher with 2 adult children who have recently left home, one at university in the North of England.

Scenario

She was admitted 3 days previously with acute confusion secondary to mild hyponatremia and severe hypercalcemia. She was treated with intravenous fluids and pamidronate, and is well orientated and lucid.

She had a mastectomy for breast cancer 10 years ago followed by radiotherapy, but no chemotherapy. She has been seen only 6 months ago in the breast clinic and reassured that everything was ok. She has been well until this admission.

She has complained of increasing back and sacral pain and the house officer requested X-rays and prescribed NSAID which have been useful. These X-Rays have shown what appears to be bone metastases. She also has metastases on her CXR with a moderate effusion and cytology confirming malignant cells.

Your task is to explain to Mrs Hazel that she has advanced metastatic cancer and will be referred to the oncology team for further care that is likely to include chemotherapy and radiotherapy.

- You have 14 minutes until the patient/subject leaves the room followed by 1 minute for reflection before discussion with the examiners.
- Do not take the history again except for details that will help in your discussion with the patient.
- *You are not required to examine the patient/subject.*

Case 8

4.8.2 Subject Information

Role: You are Mrs Hazel, a 50 year old teacher. Your husband is retired his own building firm and you have 2 daughters who live away. The youngest is in her second year at Leeds University.

Subject definition: Patient

Scenario:
You have been told you were admitted to hospital 3 days ago having become confused at home, but you have no recollection of coming into hospital. Your main complaint is of moderately severe pain in your back and hips and also some breathlessness. You have been finding it hard to get out of bed or bend easily for several weeks, and believe that you have slipped a disc after lifting some boxes awkwardly at school. Your pain has been increasingly severe for at least the last month, but you have been too busy to see a doctor about it. It has been keeping you awake at night.

You had a left mastectomy followed by radiotherapy 10 years ago. You attend a surgical follow up clinic annually, and at your last appointment 6 months ago the registrar told you everything was OK. He examined your scar, right breast and axillae, but did not blood tests.

You believe that you are cured of cancer and do not realise that it can recur late.

You are angry that you were not told of the risk of late recurrences, and wonder why you didn't have chemotherapy 10 years ago if it was known that breast cancer could behave like this. Your response to learning that you have cancer is initially disbelief, followed by grief and then anger.

You are very keen to go home and want all your care to be as an outpatient. You want to talk to your family yourself. You have heard awful stories of chemotherapy causing hair loss and vomiting, and fear for these effects. You want to know if treatment will cure the disease, and, if now, how long you have to live. You want to plan your life and consider retiring early if the outlook is poor. You are not religious; indeed your find the thought of life after death fatuous.

Your mother died 8 years ago of a stroke, and was totally bedridden and undignified for her last 2 months of life. You are afraid of going through suffering, and wish to have your pain blotted out even if it hastens your death. You have heard about euthanasia, and would wish your life to be ended swiftly when it became too painful to continue living.

Case 8

4.8.3 Examiner Information

Problem: **Advanced metastatic breast cancer needing referral to oncology services.**

If the candidate appears to have finished early, remind them how long is left at the station and enquire if there is anything else they would like to ask, or whether they have finished. If they have finished, please allow the candidate that time for reflection and remain silent. The patient should remain until the end of the 14-minute period.

A good candidate would be expected to have agreed a summary and plan of action with the subject before closure. Nonetheless, in discussion, the examiners will usually ask the candidate (after 1 minute's reflection) to summarise the problems raised in the foregoing exchange.

The candidate should be able to explain the principles of chemotherapy and radiotherapy, with a reassurance that a reasonable period of remission might be possible. The candidate should address honestly directly questions about treatment side effects. The candidate should empathise with the patient suffering a terminal illness at a young age, and be prepared to address the fact that the cancer is likely to be incurable. The candidate should give a realistic and positive opinion about oncology care being able to offer continuing quality of life, and to tactfully defect questions about its duration to the specialist team.

The candidate should be able to deal with the patient's anger relating to the initial therapy given. The candidate should not criticise previous treatment, and even if he is notable to understand the logic of the previous therapy should still find some way of reassuring the patient about the appropriateness of previous therapy. The candidate in discussion with the examiners should be prepared to discuss the following issues:
- The pros and cons of an optimistic versus a pessimistic prognosis.
- Respect for the patient's autonomy (of which discussion should take place with the daughters and husband)
- How to address the problem of criticism of previous care of other doctors.

The candidate should be asked to identify the ethical and/or legal issues raised in this case and how they would address them. The framework for discussion should include consideration of the four underlying ethical principles:
- Respect of the patient's autonomy
- Duty to do good and not to do harm
- Duty to act justly
- Legal aspects – a detailed knowledge of medical law is *not* required.

The candidate should recognise their limit in dealing with a problem and know when, and from where, to seek further advice and support.

Candidates must demonstrate competent performance in all domains outlined in the marking schedule in order to pass this station.

4.9 Case 9
Problem: Elderly man with metastatic carcinoma of the lung.

4.9.1 Candidate Information

Role: You are the SHO on the ward. You have been asked to see the son of a patient of yours, Mr Irvine. He lives a long distance from his father and sees him only 2-3 times a year.

Please read the scenario below (you may make notes if you wish on the paper provided). When the bell sounds, enter the examination room to begin the consultation.

Subject definition: Elderly man with metastatic carcinoma of the lung

Scenario:
Mr Irvine is an elderly man with metastatic carcinoma of the lung. He is admitted with an acute episode of breathlessness and a large pleural effusion which has confirmed malignant cytology. He is very cachectic and very frail. He lives alone since his wife died 4 years ago. He claims that he has had enough and feels to unwell to undergo any further treatment. You feel that he is competent to make this decision.

Your task is to discuss Mr Irvines prognosis and decide with his son:
  i)   The idea of further investigation
  ii)   Any proposed treatment
  iii)   The likely prognosis and resuscitation status

- You have 14 minutes until the patient/subject leaves the room followed by 1 minute for reflection before discussion with the examiners.
- Do <u>not</u> take the history again except for details that will help in your discussion with the patient.
- *You are not required to examine the patient/subject.*

Case 9

4.9.2 Subject Information

Role: You are the daughter, living away from home, of Mr Joe King, aged 58 who has lung cancer and has been admitted from home.

Subject definition: patient's relative.

Scenario:
Your concern is that for the past month or two your father, Joe, has been deteriorating. You know that he has lung cancer, which has probably spread to other organs.

He lives alone after his wife died 4 years ago. He is alert and still reads the newspapers most days.

You are concerned about your father's worsening condition, and you are worried about what will happen now. What is the prognosis? How can you ensure that he will be cared for even though he has refused treatment? You are aware that he feels that he "has had enough".

Case 9

4.9.3 Examiner Information

Problem: 58 year old man with metastatic carcinoma of the lung.

If the candidate appears to have finished early, remind them how long is left at the station and enquire if there is anything else they would like to ask, or whether they have finished. If they have finished, please allow the candidate that time for reflection and remain silent. The patient should remain until the end of the 14-minute period.

A good candidate would be expected to have agreed a summary and plan of action with the subject before closure. Nonetheless, in discussion, the examiners will usually ask the candidate (after 1 minute's reflection) to summarise the problems raised in the foregoing exchange.

The candidate should be able to discuss the likely prognosis of a patient with disseminated lung cancer. The treatments and tests that might be arranged – Bronchoscopy and tissue diagnosis, possible cardio-pulmonary resuscitation – are they intrusive and what is the likelihood that they will offer any benefit?

The candidate should be asked to identify the ethical and/or legal issues raised in this case and how they would address them. The framework for discussion should include consideration of the four underlying ethical principles:

- Respect of the patient's autonomy (the patient's own competent decision that he does not want further treatment despite knowing the diagnosis
- Duty to do good and not to do harm (provide continuing, supportive care to the patient)
- Duty to act justly (respect the patient's wishes and acknowledge that investigations may be futile given the poor prognosis, but ensure that a good quality of care is maintained)
- Legal aspects – a detailed knowledge of medical law is *not* required. The patient will need to be involved in the DNR decision.

The candidate should recognise their limit in dealing with a problem and know when, and from where, to seek further advice and support.

Candidates must demonstrate competent performance in all domains outlined in the marking schedule in order to pass this station.

4.10 Case 10

Problem: **Commencing Warfarin Treatment**

4.10.1 Candidate Information

Role: You are the thoracic medicine SHO.

Please read the scenario below. You may make notes on the paper provided. When the bell sounds, enter the examination room.

Subject definition: Patient with a pulmonary embolus

Scenario:
You have just been phoned by the Nuclear Medicine department to say that a V/Q scan on a 35 year old women gives a high probability of pulmonary embolism. Your task is to explain the diagnosis, and the need for treatment with Warfarin. You should give the patient appropriate information to take this drug safely.

- You have 14 minutes until the patient/subject leaves the room followed by 1 minute for reflection before discussion with the examiners.
- Do not take the history again except for details that will help in your discussion with the patient.
- You are not required to examine the patient/subject.

Case 10

4.10.2 Subject Information

Role: You are Julie Collins, who are about to be told you have a blood clot on the lung

Subject definition: Patient

Scenario:
You are a 35 year old marketing manager who developed sudden onset left sided chest pain and breathlessness 2 days after returning from a business trip. You are obviously concerned that this could represent "economy class" syndrome although do not know much more than you have read in the papers.

You do not know how this is treated and generally dislike taking tablets. However you are taking St John's Wort for mild depression. You fly at least once a month for work, and your job depends on being able to travel. You also play squash once a week and take occasional aspirin for strains after a game.

You live with a long term partner and were planning to start a family in the next few months.

Case 10

4.10.3 Examiner Information

Problem: Pulmonary embolus requiring Warfarin treatment.

If the candidate appears to have finished early, remind them how long is left at the station and enquire if there is anything else they would like to ask, or whether they have finished. If they have finished, please allow the candidate that time for reflection and remain silent. The patient should remain until the end of the 14-minute period.

A good candidate would be expected to have agreed a summary and plan of action with the subject before closure. Nonetheless, in discussion, the examiners will usually ask the candidate (after 1 minute's reflection) to summarise the problems raised in the foregoing exchange.

The candaidate should be able to explain the diagnosis of PE and elicit risk factors for this condition. The candidate should be able to explain the need for treatment and the precautions needed. The candidate would be expected to obtain all information needed to treat safely including relevant past medical history, drug history and lifestyle factors that would impact on taking warfarin.

The candidate should be able give adequate information to the patient on how to take the treatment and what precautions to observe, in terms suitable for a patient to understand.

The candidate should recognise their limit in dealing with a problem and know when, and from where, to seek further advice and support.
Candidates must demonstrate competent performance in all domains outlined in the marking schedule in order to pass this station.

4.11 Case 11

Problem: Diabetic patient needing to start dialysis

4.11.1   Candidate Information:

Role: You are the Endocrine SHO in diabetic clinic.

Please read the scenario below. You may make notes on the paper provided. When the bell sounds, enter the examination room.

Subject definition: Mr Jones, a 66 year old man with type 2 Diabetes Mellitus.

Scenario:
Mr Jones is a 66 year old man who has had diabetes for 10 years, treated with oral hypoglycaemic agents. He has had nephropathy for 6 years and his creatanine has been rising. It is now 350. Please discuss the situation and the options regarding renal replacement therapy to determine if dialysis would be appropriate.

You are not expected to make the final decision as to further treatment, as he will be referred to a nephrologist.

- You have 14 minutes until the patient/subject leaves the room followed by 1 minute for reflection before discussion with the examiners.
- Do <u>not</u> take the history again except for details that will help in your discussion with the patient.
- *You are not required to examine the patient/subject.*

Case 11

4.11.2   Subject Information

Role: You are Mr Jones a 66 year old with diabetes. You are attending for your 6 monthly review appointment. You did a urine test a few weeks ago.

Subject definition: Patient

Scenario:
You are a 66 year old man who has had diabetes for about 10 years for which you take tablets. You are also on medication for blood pressure and know that the diabetes has affected the kidneys although you are unsure of the significance of this. Your diabetic control is not that good as you find it difficult to stick to a diet. Your BMs are usually over 10.

Recently you have noticed that your ankles are quite swollen and you get breathless on walking any distance uphill. You also feel very tired and have an annoying itch. You do not, as far as you know have any other medical problems.

You retired on health grounds aged 59 and live with your wife. You are still able to drive, although your wife has to push the trolley when you go to the supermarket. Your main social activity is going to the Pub two nights a week when you enjoy 2 or 3 pints of beer. You do not drink spirits. You smoke 10 a day having cut down from 40 a day. You like a fried breakfast although you know it is not good for you.

Your wife is in good health.

You do not know anyone that has been on dialysis although you know the last hospital fete was to raise money for a dialysis machine, but you do not know much about what it entails.

Case 11

4.11.3   Examiner Information

Problem: **Diabetic patient needing to start dialysis.**
If the candidate appears to have finished early, remind them how long is left at the station and enquire if there is anything else they would like to ask, or whether they have finished.   If they have finished, please allow the candidate that time for reflection and remain silent. The patient should remain until the end of the 14-minute period.

A good candidate would be expected to have agreed a summary and plan of action with the subject before closure.   Nonetheless, in discussion, the examiners will usually ask the candidate (after 1 minute's reflection) to summarise the problems raised in the foregoing exchange.

The candidate should be able to explain to the patient that his kidneys are not working and why. They should be able to explain the significance of this and what would happen in left untreated. This should be done in an emphatic manner in terms the patient will be able to understand, avoiding technical terms.

The candidate should be able to ascertain the current level of functioning and quality of life of the patient in a sensitive way, to determine the appropriateness of dialysis. The candidate should then be able to go on to find out the patients current understanding of dialysis and explain the different types of renal replacement therapy in simple terms to the patient.

The candidate would **not** be expected to come to a final decision if renal replacement therapy is to be started.

The candidate should recognise their limit in dealing with a problem and know when, and from where, to seek further advice and support.

Candidates must demonstrate competent performance in all domains outlined in the marking schedule in order to pass this station.

4.12 Case 12

Scenario   **A Jehovah's Witness with a Stroke**

4.12.1   Candidate Information

Role: You are the medical SHO on call. You have just seen Mr Joyes in A&E and are now about to talk to his daughter.

Please read the scenario below. You may make notes on the paper provided. When the bell sounds, enter the examination room.

Subject definition: Daughter of patient

Scenario

Mr Joyes is a 63 year old gentleman. He has been on Warfarin treatment for 4 months after having been found to be in AF. He has been admitted with a headache and a right hemiparesis. After arriving at A&E his conscious level deteriorated and a CT scan revealed a haemorrhagic stroke. He is a Jehovah's Witness. Please discuss his further management with his daughter. His INR is 3.6

- You have 14 minutes until the patient/subject leaves the room followed by 1 minute for reflection before discussion with the examiners.
- Do <u>not</u> take the history again except for details that will help in your discussion with the patient.
- *You are not required to examine the patient/subject.*

Case 12

4.12.2   Subject Information

Role: You are the daughter of Mr Joyes who has just been bought into A&E after suffering a stroke

Subject definition: Patient's daughter

Scenario:
Your father has been bought to hospital as an emergency today. He complained of a headache this morning and then the right side of his face went droopy. He was unable to stand. Since coming into hospital he has deteriorated and is now unconscious.

He has been fairly well all his life with no major illnesses. He is fit and active and is very active in his church (he is a Jehovah's Witness). However a few months ago he saw his GP because of some palpitations and was found to be in fibrillation. His GP recommended that he start warfarin to prevent strokes. He has been on this for four months and has religiously been attending the anticoagulation clinic.

Your father is a strict Jehovah's Witness and would not want any blood transfusions or blood products even if his life was in danger.

Case 12

4.12.3 Examiner Information

Problem: A Jehovah's Witness with a Stroke

If the candidate appears to have finished early, remind them how long is left at the station and enquire if there is anything else they would like to ask, or whether they have finished. If they have finished, please allow the candidate that time for reflection and remain silent. The patient should remain until the end of the 14-minute period.

A good candidate would be expected to have agreed a summary and plan of action with the subject before closure. Nonetheless, in discussion, the examiners will usually ask the candidate (after 1 minute's reflection) to summarise the problems raised in the foregoing exchange.

A candidate should be able to explain the diagnosis and how the warfarin may have contributed to this and go on to explain the benefits of reversing the warfarin. The candidate should be able to explain the possible treatments for this including FFP and vitamin K, including the benefits of each but also explain that FFP is a blood product.

The candidates should recognise the legal and ethical principles of autonomy to refuse even lifesaving treatments and the circumstances where this applies. The candidate should be sensitive about others religious beliefs.

The candidate should recognise their limit in dealing with a problem and know when, and from where, to seek further advice and support.

Candidates must demonstrate competent performance in all domains outlined in the marking schedule in order to pass this station.

4.13 Case 13

Scenario: **Consent to an HIV treatment**

4.13.1   Candidate Information

Role: You are a medical SHO seeing a young lady admitted last night with a sore throat. You have a clinical suspicion of HIV seroconversion.

Please read the scenario below. You may make notes on the paper provided. When the bell sounds, enter the examination room.

Subject definition: Miss Jones, the patients

Scenario:
You have admitted Miss Jones, a 22 year old student nurse who has a sore throat and a rash. You have a clinical suspicion of HIV seroconversion. Please discuss this with her and counsel her regarding an HIV test.

- You have 14 minutes until the patient/subject leaves the room followed by 1 minute for reflection before discussion with the examiners.
- Do not take the history again except for details that will help in your discussion with the patient.
- *You are not required to examine the patient/subject.*

Case 13

4.13.2   Subject Information

Role: You are Miss Jones a 22 year old student nurse who attended hospital with a rash and sore throat.

Subject definition: Patient

Scenario:
You are a 22 year old student nurse, who has just started the clinical phase of the course. You have been feeling unwell for two weeks with a sore throat and fevers. You have noticed some glands up in your neck, and yesterday developed a widespread rash with blotchy red lesions. You saw your GP who has sent you to casualty for further tests.

You drink 4 pints of lager each day over the weekend and one day during the week on average. You smoke 15 a day and occasionally smoke cannabis. You have once tried cocaine a few months ago, but have never injected drugs. You have a regular boyfriend who you have protected sex with, you are not on the pill. You also met a Nigerian man at a party two months ago and had unprotected sex with him – you have not told your boyfriend about this. You have not stayed in touch with this man, but have his mobile phone number. You have never had a blood transfusion. Your last holiday was to visit your parents in Ireland. Last summer you went to Majorca and have travelled to Florida previously.

You are obviously concerned as to what is wrong. You thought you had 'flu but cannot shake it off – the ward manager where you are having your first attachment is complaining about the time you have taken off and says you may fail your attachment.

Case 13

4.13.3   Examiner Information

PROBLEM: CONSENT FOR AN HIV TEST

If the candidate appears to have finished early, remind them how long is left at the station and enquire if there is anything else they would like to ask, or whether they have finished.   If they have finished, please allow the candidate that time for reflection and remain silent. The patient should remain until the end of the 14-minute period.

A good candidate would be expected to have agreed a summary and plan of action with the subject before closure.   Nonetheless, in discussion, the examiners will usually ask the candidate (after 1 minute's reflection) to summarise the problems raised in the foregoing exchange.

The candidate should take a brief history of the current illness as an introduction to the issue and explore risk factors for HIV infection so as to go on to sensitively introduce HIV infection as a possible diagnosis. This needs to be done in a non-judgmental manner.

The candidate should be able to discuss the implications of a positive test including who to tell and implications on further training as a nurse.

The candidate should be able to discuss issues regarding informing boyfriend and understand the legal situations where confidence could be breached.

The candidate should recognise their limit in dealing with a problem and know when, and from where, to seek further advice and support.

Candidates must demonstrate competent performance in all domains outlined in the marking schedule in order to pass this station.

4.14 Case 14

Scenario: Starting steroids in Rheumatoid Arthritis

4.14.1 Candidate Information

Role: You are the Rheumatology SHO in outpatients. You have just discussed the case of Mrs Davies with your consultant and he feels she should start steroids. Please discuss this with her.

Please read the scenario below. You may make notes on the paper provided. When the bell sounds, enter the examination room.

Scenario:
Mrs Davies is a 36 year old women who has had Rheumatoid Arthritis for 3 years. So far her main symptom has been stiff hands and has required only NSAIDS to control her symptoms. However over the last few months she has had worsening disease and you feel she needs to start Prednisolone to control her symptoms. Please discuss this with her.

- You have 14 minutes until the patient/subject leaves the room followed by 1 minute for reflection before discussion with the examiners.
- Do <u>not</u> take the history again except for details that will help in your discussion with the patient.
- You are not expected to examine the patient/subject

Case 14

4.14.2   Subject Information

Role: You are Mrs Davies a 36 year old lady who suffers from Rheumatoid Arthritis.

Subject definition: Patient

Scenario:
You were devastated when first diagnosed with Rheumatoid Arthritis 3 years ago but have slowly come to terms with it, especially as you have not had to take regular medication. However you have become increasingly concerned recently as your symptoms have started to worsen. Your hands are very stiff first thing in the morning and you are finding it difficult to prepare breakfast for your children. You are also finding it difficult to walk because of pain in your feet.

You work in a hairdressers and are expected to take care of your appearance for work. You have two children aged 3 and 6. The older had chicken pox last year but you have never suffered from it. Your mother suffers from osteoporosis and had a hip fracture last year. Your father had a heart attack aged 50 and died of a stroke in his sixties.

You are concerned about having to take steroids. You know they make you put on weight and make your face look fat which concerns you with your work. You are also worried about getting infections from your children. In general you prefer to avoid taking tablets – you have tried several herbal treatments for your arthritis.

Case 14

4.14.3 Examiner Information

Problem: Starting steroids in Rheumatoid Arthritis.

If the candidate appears to have finished early, remind them how long is left at the station and enquire if there is anything else they would like to ask, or whether they have finished. If they have finished, please allow the candidate that time for reflection and remain silent. The patient should remain until the end of the 14-minute period. A good candidate would be expected to have agreed a summary and plan of action with the subject before closure. Nonetheless, in discussion, the examiners will usually ask the candidate (after 1 minute's reflection) to summarise the problems raised in the foregoing exchange.

The candidate should be able to explore the impact of RA on the patients daily activities and quality of life and explain the need for further treatment and advantages of using steroids. They should also be able to explain the side effects of steroids and explain the risks of infections especially chicken pox.

The candidate must be able to adequately and clearly explain that the patient must not stop taking without medical supervision and make sure she knows what to do should she become unwell.

The candidate should recognise their limit in dealing with a problem and know when, and from where, to seek further advice and support.

Candidates must demonstrate competent performance in all domains outlined in the marking schedule in order to pass this station.

4.15 Case 15

Problem: Pre pregnancy counselling post fetal loss due to poor glycaemic control

4.15.1   Candidate Information

Role: You are the SHO in diabetic clinic. You are seeing a new patient who has been referred by the hospital obstetrician.

Please read the scenario below (you may make notes if you wish on the paper provided).   When the bell sounds, enter the examination room to begin the consultation.

Subject definition: SHO in clinic

Scenario:

Dear Doctor,

Thank you for seeing this 28 year old lady who has suffered from type 1 diabetes since the age of 9.

She had a spontaneous pregnancy at the age of 22 and delivered prematurely at 36 weeks gestation as a result of pre eclampsia. Her daughter was diagnosed with a coarctation of the aorta during fetal echocardiography but had this corrected during infancy.

She has recently suffered a miscarriage at 22 weeks probably as a result of her poor glycaemic control, autopsy revealed several severe congenital malformations.

She is very upset and is in need of further diabetic education.

She does not seem to want to take any responsibility for her control and would like to get pregnant again.

Her HbA1c has never been less than 11% and her attendance to our clinics has been very poor even during her preganacy.

I'd be grateful for your assistance

Best wishes

Dr Howard

- You have 14 minutes until the patient/subject leaves the room followed by 1 minute for reflection before discussion with the examiners.
- Do <u>not</u> take the history again except for details that will help in your discussion with the patient.
- *You are not required to examine the patient/subject*

Case 15

4.15.2   Subject Information

Role: Miss Brewer 28 year old lady

Scenario:
You have had type 1 diabetes since you were 8

You have had to inject yourself with insulin for many years and have got fed up of coming to hospitals as you seem to have spent your entire childhood in clinics

Your daughter, aged 6, had a congenital abnormality of the heart requiring major surgery. It nearly destroyed you watching what she had to go through, spending weeks lying on a camp bed at her bedside in Great hospital. You were told it was possibly caused by the diabetes but were never given any other advice. It was only after a recent horrible miscarriage were you told that you had to sort out your diabetes

You feel very guilty but at the same time very angry that no one actually gave you concrete advice about this. If it was so bad, why did the diabetic clinic not contact you?

You are eager to have your sugars controlled but initially feel it is the doctor's responsibility.

You eventually agree that it is a partnership and agree to comply with re-education, monitoring and abstaining from further pregnancy until your control has improved.

Case 15

4.15.3   Examiner information

- Pre-conceptual counselling should not be confused with antenatal care.
- Pre-conceptual counselling has several components:
  - It begins with attitudes and practices that value pregnant women, children, and families and respects the diversity of people's lives and experiences.
  - It incorporates informed choice, thus encouraging women and men to understand health issues that may affect conception and pregnancy.
  - It encourages women and men to prepare actively for pregnancy, and enables them to be as healthy as possible.
  - It attempts to identify couples who are at increased risk of producing babies with a genetic malformation, and provide them with sufficient knowledge to make informed decisions.

The candidate should:
  - Approach this in a blame free, non-confrontational manner
  - Sympathise with the patients loss
  - Establish what the problems are regarding glycaemic control
  - Establish any education that took place after first birth
  - Recommend that she does not get pregnant again until her control is improved to reduce risks to herself and the foetus
  - Agree that she will need to be seen frequently by the DSN and diabetes team for education and control
  - Try to establish a partnership

Diabetes guidelines

- **Refer to a specialist and, if available, to a diabetic preconceptual counselling clinic.**

- **Poor control of diabetes** increases the risks of major congenital abnormality and spontaneous abortion. A normal glycosylated haemoglobin level at the onset of pregnancy appears to reduce this risk [Super et al, 1986].

- There is no evidence that metformin or the sulphonylureas are teratogenic. However, metformin may be associated with growth retardation and hyperbilirubinaemia. Sulphonylureas cross the placenta and may cause hyperinsulinaemia and macrosomia in the fetus) [Seymour and Pugh, 2000; American Diabetes Association, 2003].

- It is very important to optimize glycaemic control pre-conceptually, as the rate of major congenital abnormalities can be reduced if control is good in the first 8 weeks of pregnancy [Diabetes UK, 2000]. Aim for a glycosylated haemoglobin level of not more than 1% above the upper limit of normal. Effective contraception should be used until this target is achieved [American Diabetes Association, 2003].

- Following hospital review, in the ideal situation all women should be switched to human insulin. However, in certain cases the specialist may decide that metformin is an acceptable alternative for the pre-conceptual period

4.15.4   Tutorial: Diabetes in Pregnancy

Diabetes in pregnancy poses numerous problems for both mother and foetus but the outcome has improved because of the emphasis on excellent glycaemic control and preconception counselling. A normal pregnancy is associated with insulin resistance through the effects of human placental lactogen and progesterone. The effect is pronounced in the late second and third trimesters.   This is thought to favour nutrient transfer to the foetus because as the postprandial blood glucose level rises, there is compensatory hyperinsulinaemia and lipolysis is enhanced.

- In pregnant women with pre-existing diabetes, glycaemic control tends to worsen and insulin requirements will usually double in comparison to pre-pregnancy values.
- Maternal diabetes is associated with various foetal developmental malformations, including an increased risk of spina bifida, sacral agenesis, cleft palate, renal agenesis, ureteric duplication, anorectal atresia.
- The incidence of spontaneous abortion is directly related to the HbA1C value. One study demonstrated foetal loss due to miscarriage of 9% in diabetic pregnancies that were well controlled in comparison to 29% in those with poor control.
- Another associated problem with poor glycaemic control, is accelerated foetal growth due to increased delivery of glucose and other nutrients. This is secondary to fetal hyperinsulinaemia, which provokes nutrient storage. Large gestational age infants are twice as common in diabetic as in non-diabetic problems, with the associated problems of birth trauma, hypoglycaemia and hypocalcaemia.
- Management of pregnancy in diabetic women with Type 1 Diabetes Mellitus should start with pre-conceptional counselling, with special emphasis on tightening glycaemic control attempting to achieve fasting blood glucose levels of <6mmol/l and postprandial peaks of <8.0mmol/l. In view of the increased risk of neural tube defects, it is essential to start Folic Acid supplementation at 5mg per day in the pre-conception stage.
- During pregnancy itself, patients should be seen every two weeks, until 34 weeks gestation and then weekly.
- Pregnancies are also associated with worsening of diabetic microvascular disease, particularly nephropathy and retinopathy. With respect to diabetic nephropathy, blood pressure control should be meticulous with Methyldopa and/or Nifedipine (SR or LA preparations only). Aim for a BP <140/90.
- Diabetic retinopathy especially pre-proliferative and proliferative retinopathy, may deteriorate rapidly during pregnancy, this is often a consequence of very poor glycaemic control, or a rapid improvement in glycaemic control. There is no contra-indication to photo-coagulation during pregnancy.
- Other important complications of diabetic pregnancy include pre-eclampsia which is at least double the rate in the non-diabetic pregnancy. In cases where early delivery is required, Dexamethasone may be needed to hasten fetal lung maturation. Dexamethasone treatment is usually associated with deterioration in glycaemic control. Insulin dose will need to be increased.
- During labour, diabetes is controlled by intravenous infusions of insulin and glucose in most cases. The glucose/insulin/potassium infusion regime is suitable.
- Newborn babies of poorly controlled diabetic women are often macrosomic with hyperglycaemic, polycythaemia and an increased risk of respiratory distress syndrome.

- Gestational diabetes is diabetes that is first diagnosed during pregnancy. There are no diagnostic criteria that are widely accepted. Locally any abnormality in the GTT is deemed gestational diabetes mellitus.
- Who to screen regularly by glycosuria testing or even a formal GTT at 24-28 gestation: consider re-checking the GTT at 32-34 gestation.
- Glycosuria
    - Previous Gestational Diabetes Mellitus
    - Family history of diabetes
    - Previous macrosomic baby
    - Previous Stillbirth
    - Obesity
    - Polyhydramnios
    - Large for gestational age
- If a mother has glycosuria it should be repeated 3-7 days. If positive proceed to GTT. Another accepted definition is the WHO definition, which states that a plasma glucose 7mmol/l or greater or a 120 min value of 7.8 mmol/l or greater should be considered as gestational diabetes. A random sample alone may suffice. The management of gestational diabetes is initially with strict dietary control. If glycaemic control deteriorates with glucose levels about 8.0mmol/l then insulin treatment is required, which is the case of 10 - 30% of GDM pregnancies.
- The lifetime risk of developing Diabetes in women with GDM is 30%.
- In pregnancy, one should aim for a HbA1C of <6.5% and preferably <6.0%. HbA1c% is checked every two weeks in pregnancy.

Relative Risk of Congenital Malformation versus HbA1% as an Index of Glycaemic Control

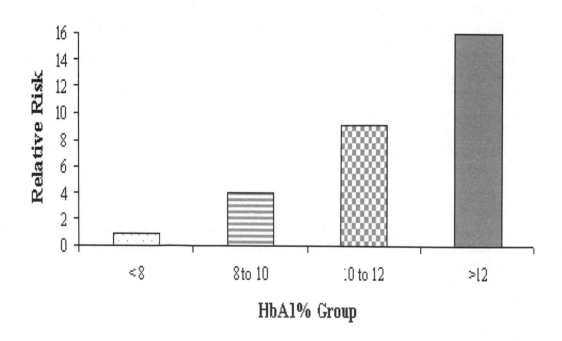

5 MEDICAL ETHICS

5.1 *Introduction*

Good medical practice is based on a combination of moral and political enterprises. As a practising doctor you will need to make the best possible decisions regarding patient care. In making these decisions, you will often ask yourself:

- What can be done for this patient?
- What should be done?
- What can I do to ensure that what should be done can be done for my patient?

Patients must be able to trust doctors with their lives and well beings.
To justify that trust the medical profession has a duty to maintain a good standard of practice and care and show respect for human life. A doctor's training therefore needs to cover not only the scientific and technical aspects of medicine but also the analysis and the understanding of relevant ethical issues and moral dilemmas.

Good Medical Practice:
All patients irrespective of race, gender and social class are entitled to good standards of care from their doctors. The essential tenets of good practice directed at medical ethics are as follows:-

- Professional competence
- Good Relationships with Patients and Colleagues
- Thinking Ethically when making decisions regarding your patients and colleagues

5.1.1 Professional competence

Qualities desired by the GMC

A practising doctor must be competent at making suitable decisions and taking prompt action when necessary. This includes adequate assessment of the patient's condition through history taking and clinical examination, providing and arranging investigations and treatment as necessary, and referring the patient to another practitioner when indicated.

Whilst providing care a doctor must at all times recognise the limits of his own professional competence and be willing to consult colleagues as appropriate without delay.

Record keeping

It is in everyone's interests if the doctor or health care professional keeps clear and accurate patient records, which report:

- All relevant clinical findings
- The subsequent decisions made
- Information given to patients regarding their condition
- Investigations requested
- Clear documentation of any drugs prescribed or treatment initiated and when this treatment was administered
- Clear accounts should of any untoward reaction to either a drug prescribed, investigative procedure, and treatment.

Personal development

Professional competence can only be maintained if you, as a doctor, invest in the standard of your practice by keeping up to date with your knowledge and skills throughout your working life. You should also be prepared to learn new skills as directed by your speciality of interest.

Furthermore, doctors must work closely with their colleagues to monitor and improve the quality of care provided .We should all be aware of medical practices governed by law.

5.1.2 Good Relationships with Patients and Colleagues

Patients

A doctor should respect the patient's privacy and dignity at all times.

Successful relationships between doctors and patients are built upon trust

It is the doctor's duty to establish and maintain that trust by making the care of the patient his first concern. Doctors are actively encouraged to listen to patients and to respect their views, as well as to address patients politely and considerately. Patients have a right to ask questions relating to their condition, its treatment and prognosis. It is a doctor's duty to furnish the patient with this information in a way that is comprehensive to the patient.

Furthermore a doctor must respect the right of a patient to be fully involved in the decisions about their care and also respect the right of a patient to refuse treatment or to refuse to take part in clinical teaching or research.

Doctors themselves are human beings and may have rigid views about various aspects of life. A practising doctor must however not allow his views about a patient's lifestyle, culture, beliefs, race, colour, sex, sexuality, age, social status to prejudice medical consultations or the treatment that is given to the patient. If a practising doctor feels that his own beliefs might affect the treatment that he is able to provide a patient. It is his duty to explain this to the patient and inform them of their right to see another doctor. Furthermore, treatment should not be refused or delayed, even if the patient's actions may have contributed to their condition, or because their clinical condition may be putting the doctor at risk.

If the trust between a doctor and patient breaks down, it is possible that either party may wish to end the relationship. Should this occur, it is the duty of the doctor to do his best to make sure that arrangements are made promptly for the continuing care of the patient. Patient records and other relevant information should be made available without delay to the new doctor.

Patients have a right to expect that any personal information, which they disclose during the course of a doctor/patient relationship, will not be passed on without their consent. In some exceptional circumstances, it may be in the best interests of the public if some patient information is passed on, although the doctor will need to act responsibly within the boundaries of medical legalities. It must be added that doctors should never in the course of their practice abuse their professional position to either establish improper relationships with patients and their close relatives, or to put pressure on patients to gain financial or other benefits.

Doctors and their colleagues

Rarely, a doctor may become suspicious that colleagues' conduct, performance or health is a threat to the patient's interests. In this situation, the doctor should exercise responsibility and honesty to establish the essential facts and then notify someone from the employing authority or from a regulatory body. If uncertainty does arise, it is reasonable to ask the advice of an experienced colleague in a confidential manner. This will allow for any uncertainty to be investigated in a blame free culture where lessons can be learned by all. The safety of the patient must however come first at all times.

Similarly, a practising doctor, you may find that you yourself, falls victim to a serious communicable condition or other illness which may affect both your clinical judgement and performance. In this situation, advice from a consultant in Occupational Health or another suitably qualified colleague should be taken to establish in what ways medical practice should be modified. In this situation, a doctor should not rely on his own assessment of the risk to patients.

As with patients, doctors should not discriminate against colleagues, including doctors applying the post, because of differing views on lifestyle, culture, beliefs, race, colour, sex, sexuality or age. Furthermore, a doctor should never make any patient doubt a colleague's knowledge or skills by making unnecessary or unsustainable comments about these colleagues.

Doctors in multidisciplinary teams

Health-care, is increasingly provided by multidisciplinary teams. Doctors are expected to work constructively within such teams and to respect the skills and contributions of colleagues within that team. As a doctor leading a team, it is your duty to make sure that the whole team understands the need to provide a polite and effective service, and to treat patient information as confidential. Disagreements can and do arise, and in this situation, solutions to difficult decisions should be found where the quality of patient care is the final determinant.

5.1.3 Thinking ethically

Factors that question individual ethical values cannot always be answered by simply applying the rules of good medical practice. There are a number of reasons for this. First and foremost, it is unlikely that all properly informed people will agree on the right action for a given specific situation. If we are to practise medicine in a way we think is right, we must first appreciate that:

- No two clinical scenarios will be identical. For each situation, the doctor should clarify the facts to each specific situation and be aware of all the relevant issues.
- Care should be taken to ensure that all arguments put forward, are logical.
- All views should be consistent and subject too critical analysis.
- There should be willingness to adapt or change views in the light of such analysis in a legal framework.

Valued judgements:

Just as scientific evidence should be properly evaluated, good medical practice also relies upon problems that have been properly analysed and assessed with a making of valued judgements.

Clinical Judgement:
We as doctors are familiar with clinical judgements. This is an attribute exercised by the experienced clinician in resolving a diagnostic or therapeutic dilemma. It derives from the blend of formal training, knowledge acquired from the medical literature and above all clinical experience.

Moral judgement:
Valued judgements are made in relation to moral values. Such judgement is "difficult" (Hippocrates), "mysterious" and irreducible (Kant).

Moral, like *clinical judgement* involves discerning what evidence is relevant, reviewing it and coming to a conclusion whose rightness may be evident, if ever only in retrospect.

Conflicts:
Individuals or groups may give different ordering or priorities to particular moral values, which may lead to rational individuals making radically different choices in similar circumstances.

These differing views are often, in this context referred to as *conflicts*.

Conflict is often the origin of important ethical issues. In most situations, it is seen as vital and enduring and for this reason many scenario's you are examined will be based on a conflict of thinking and reasoning. The importance of making these conflicts explicit is that a group in which differing individuals are explicitly "taking care" of different values may be more effective than one which is not.

Avoiding conflict at all costs will entail, usually continuous compromise, which would be unacceptable to most situations encountered. On the other hand, conflict itself, without valued reasoning, can cause major harm.

As a doctor, you must be able to and be prepared to justify your decisions and actions with regard to both an evidential scientific basis and the ethical values in the process of decision-making.

5.1.4 Ethical values and patient care
In dealing with your case scenario's in the examination, you must be able to communicate your argument with relation to the four important ethical principles. The examiner will expect you to have an understanding of these. They are:
- Autonomy
- Beneficence
- Non-maleficence
- Justice

Respect for patient autonomy:
Autonomy literally means "self-rule". It is the capacity to think, decide and act on the basis of such thought and decision, freely and independently. Respect for patient autonomy requires that health professionals (and others, including the patient's family) help patients make their own decisions (e.g. by providing important information), and respect to follow those decisions (even when the health professional believes the patient's decision is wrong).

Beneficence (promotion of what is best for the patient):

This principle emphasises the moral importance of doing good to others (particularly, in the medical context, doing good to patients). It entails doing what is best for the patient, and raises the question of who should be the judge of what is best. The principle of beneficence is often interpreted as focusing on what an objective assessment by a relevant health professional would determine as in the patient's best interests. The patient's own views are captured by the principle of respect for patient autonomy.

In most situations, respect for the principle of beneficence and for the principle of respect for patient autonomy lead to the same conclusion, because most of the time patients want what is (objectively) in their best interests. The two principles conflict when a competent patient chooses a course of action that is not in his or her best interests.

Non- maleficence (avoiding harm):

This principle states that we should not harm patients. In most situations, it does not add anything useful to the principle of beneficence. Most treatments carry some risk of doing more harm than good, but it does not follow that such treatments should be avoided on the grounds that avoiding harming a patient takes priority over doing good. Rather, the potential good and harms and their probabilities must be weighted up to decide what, overall, is in the patient's best interests. The main reason for retaining the principle of non-maleficence is that it is generally thought that we have a *prima facie* duty not to harm anyone, whereas we owe a duty of beneficence to a limited number of people only.

Justice:

A prima facie moral obligation to be just or fair is a common feature of many moral theories. Aristotle's formal analysis of obligation of justice is common to many different substantive accounts of justice. This theory requires equals to be treated equally and unequal's to be treated unequally in relation to morally relevant inequalities.

Time and resources do not allow every patient the best possible treatment. Health professionals have to decide how much time to spend with different patients, and decisions must be made about limitations on the treatments that can be offered at various levels with a health care system. The principle of justice emphasises 3 points.

- Patients in similar situations should normally have access to similar health care.
- When determining what level of health care should be available for one set of patients, we must take into account the effect of such a use of resources on other patients. In other words, we must try to distribute limited resources (time, money intensive care beds) fairly. This decision will be based upon the relative needs of the patients.
- Distribution should be such that it maximises beneficial outcomes
- Distribution should avoid waste of scarce resources
- Distribution should be such that it provides equality of access to health care

We must accept the rights of a patient to have access to a good quality of care.

5.1.5 Ethical Theories

5.1.5.1 Consequentialism:

These are moral theories (notably *Utilitarianism*) maintain that the results of the actions (or of rules for action) are what matter.

This ethical approach is often based on choosing a moral action which will maximise utility or happiness of the greatest number and minimise misery. The right action in any situation is that which, all possible actions considered, leads to the maximum sum of human happiness (where happiness is positive and misery is negative)

It was developed by two British philosophers: John Stuart Mill (in a more qualitative form) and Jeremy Bentham (in a more quantitative form). Hence the utilitarianism maxim, "Promoting the greatest happiness for the greatest number".

However, certain dilemmas may arise:
– Which consequences are likely to arise as a result of the action
– And if so, are the probabilities, likely, possible or remote?
– Are the consequences going to affect the individual, population or environment?
– Who will evaluate will these observations and by what means?

Practical problems include unintended side effects and focussing on the measurable. Furthermore, in many instances, you might be faced with several possible causes of action that you could take for any one given problem. The question arises then, which is the right course of action to take? In accordance with consequentialism, the way to deal with this question is to consider the consequences of each of the possible causes of action considered. The right action is the one that has the best foreseeable consequences. It is only the foreseeable consequences that are ethically important. Alone, consequentialism is not a complete moral theory because it does not focus on the aspects of the consequences that are morally important. The utilitarian aspect of the consequences relies upon moral theory.

Felicific Calculus
Felicific Calculus, otherwise known as a calculus of happiness, is the summation of total happiness and total misery. This quantification of happiness was put forward by Bentham and it has evolved further to become a concept and a quality adjusted life years (QUALY) which has been used in healthcare prioritisation.

5.1.5.2 Deontological - or Duty Based – Ethics

Deontology (From Greek for "what is dew"
These are theories of:
– Rights
– Duties
– Or of what is absolutely right or wrong (as opposed to relatively good and bad) to do.
– Theories are based upon unconditional respect for all forms of life

The philosopher that developed this theory was actually a German called Emmanuel Kant. This theory was based on a reason that has been enormously influential. In this theory the question Which action is right? is answered by considering, not the consequences of the possible actions, but rather the nature of the actions themselves. This means we should take into account fundamentalised values such as a duty to respect each other in our mutual dealings. One example of this type is that we should not lie to each other. The consequentialist however would ask Would telling the truth or telling a lie bring about the best consequences? In contrast, a duty-based emphasis would argue that, even if lying has a better consequence, it remains morally wrong to lie.

5.1.6 Ethical Theories in Medical Practice
Doctors tend to take elements from both ethical theories for decision making.

For example most individuals believe that it can be wrong to tell a lie, even in circumstances when telling a lie might have the best consequences, but also believe that there are times when the consequences of telling the truth are so much worse than telling a lie that it would be right to lie. An important area of medicine, where it is helpful to think about fundamental moral beliefs is the question of confidentiality. Both theories suggested rely on a high standard of medical confidentiality. These however may become conflicting when a doctor knows something about the patient that the patient wants to keep confidential. An example of this type is a man who is HIV positive but does not want his wife to know. For utilitarian's, the main issue is the consequences of breaching or not breaching confidentiality. All possible consequences must be considered, including the effects that breaching patient confidentiality will have on the patient and spouse, and maybe effects more generally on patients' trust in doctors and the possible demise of the doctor-patient relationship. For duty based ethics there is a further key issue: this is the morality of breaching confidentiality, independently of any consideration of consequences.

Applying moral theory or principals does not always get very far in solving an ethical problem or resolving a disagreement. One of the problems faced is the lack of a clear and comprehensive definition or explanation of key terms required for conceptual analysis. For example, in a debate regarding abortion, all parties may agree that it is wrong to kill a person. One of the disputes in this area is whether a foetus under the age of 12 weeks is in fact a person. It is important for the decision-maker to be properly informed of the pros and cons of the possible decisions are weighed up prior to taking the lead on the chosen decision.

5.1.7 Consistency

What is consistency?
In logic, a group of statements is consistent if they could all be true together.

No single medical situation is going to be entirely the same. Specific cases however have the fundamental ruling moral argument. Ethics is not so rigid that principles are carved in stone. There is flexibility to give each situation unique thought processes so as to provide a tailor made solution. It is not possible to simply look at a situation and decide whether we believe it to be morally right or wrong. We need to explore the full implications of the situation as actual specific situations. In practice then if a principle has implications for specific situations that we believe are clearly wrong, the principle must either be rejected or modified. Each argument put forward must have logical connotations. It is improper and unethical to react on one's gut reaction as there is no ethical argument or justification of raw reaction. Each situation requires ethical reasoning which itself is an interactive process involving consideration in individual situations and application of general principles. Fundamental logical requisite is consistency. If what you believe is right for one situation but seems inconsistent with what you believe is right in another situation you must either identify a morally relevant difference between the two situations or change your views. Comparison of the problematic situation with other less contentious situations is one of the most powerful ways of considering a difficult issue in medical ethics.

Logical Argument

To reason or to argue logically is to use a related series of statements, one of which is the conclusion and the others are the premises.

We argue from premises to a conclusion, or we support the conclusion with the premises.

It is a useful discipline to explore an argument using a valid set of questions, which would conclude to a logical solution. The basic form of logical argument is the syllogism.

If an argument is logically valid and you accept the truth of the premises, you must accept the truth of the conclusion. However you may reject the conclusion if you reject the truth of one of the premises.

5.1.8 Mistakes

Mistakes in reasoning are called "fallacies", and there are many typical fallacies, e.g., an argument "begs the question" if it assumes what is at stake. An example of this is "abortion must be wrong for it involves murder"

On the other hand, an argument may involve a "genetic fallacy" if it confuses the historical or psychological origin of something with its rational justification; e.g. it may be true that a patient is caused to complain because of fear or loneliness, but that is irrelevant to the question of whether the complaint is rationally justified.

5.1.9 Medical decisions

Decisions in health care must be made by all those involved: patients, doctors & nurses, family and healthcare managers. Ethical theory may not always lead to resolution of a disagreement. Two people may genuinely disagree on an ethical issue, even when they have fully considered the issues in the above ways. But if conflict is an inevitable feature of ethical analysis, how are doctors who want to practice ethical medicine going to proceed? They must take seriously the ethical dimension of decisions and must be prepared to justify publicly the decisions made and the actions taken. Such justification requires attention to both the grounds on which the decision was made and the process by which the decision was made.

Relevant questions may be as follows:-
1. Were the right people consulted in the decision making?
2. Was the decision taken in the right form?
3. Was there adequate discussion of the issues?
4. Was the decision recorded properly?
5. Was there a proper system for review of the decision?

5.2 Consent

The ethical principle that every person has a right to *self-determination* is reflected in the law through the concept of consent.

The law of governing medical practice has evolved to such an extent that medical law has become a speciality in its own right. Doctors are now subject to multiple systems of accountability. As a consequence, one clinical incident may give rise to a series of investigations, some of which may not be completed for years after the events in question. It is important that as a doctor you understand clearly your responsibilities from the outset of your career, and to keep them in mind thereafter. One aspect of medical practice is the approach a doctor takes to obtain consent from a patient regarding investigation and treatment for a given condition. The nature by which consent is obtained is not only fundamental to the patient/doctor relationship but is also a key test to the degree to which patient autonomy is respected. In order to obtain consent, the doctor discloses information to a patient who is legally competent. The patient understands the information and makes a decision voluntarily. This analysis has been incorporated into English law. For consent to treatment to be legally valid, three conditions must be satisfied.
1.   The patient must be legally competent to give (or refuse to give) consent.
2.   The patient must have sufficient information to make a choice.
3.   Consent must be given freely.

In law, it will be assumed that adult patients are competent to consent, but this assumption is rebuttable (i.e. the person challenging you on this point may be able to show that the individual in question was *not* competent, so you should always assess competency on a patient by patient basis). The competent patient must be able to:
- Comprehend the treatment information provided to him
- Believe it
- Weigh it in the balance to make an informed decision. The level of information that should be given to a patient prior to canvassing consent is a common cause of debate. Before making that decision, consider:
- The degree of risk to the patient
- The severity of the risk to the patient
- The risk to benefit ratio of the treatment
- The patient's mental state.

Although it is up to the practising doctor to decide what information should be given to the patient, this is not a licence for medical paternalism. The GMC has now issued detailed guidance on consent *"Seeking patients' consent: the ethical considerations"*, which sets out standards more demanding than current case law.

The above principles rely largely upon the provision of information. The philosophical basis of valid consent however rests upon patient autonomy. Fadden and Beauchamp, using autonomy as the basis for their analysis, proposed that informed consent should be thought of as an autonomous authorisation. According to this view, informed consent is a type of action. There is a clear distinction between consent and assent. Assent, it may be argued, is a mere submission by the patient to the doctor's authoritative order. A patient who assents does not call on his authority.

True informed consent requires that the patient does not merely assent, but specifically authorises the doctor to initiate a medical plan. Furthermore, some patients may not wish to be given a great deal of information, and may wish the doctor to make the decisions and choose the plan of management. This situation must be clearly differentiated from that of a patient who passively assents to the doctor's decision. Autonomous authorisation involves two processes. These are that the patient first assumes responsibility and then transfers it.

Consent and the law

From the legal point of view, consent provides patients with a power of veto. There are two main areas of relevant law which are battery and negligence.

Battery
This is a legal term for wrongfully touching a person, i.e. without consent.

Battery is very important for the practising doctor. Without gaining consent by the patient for a specific procedure or treatment, the doctor could be successfully sued by the patient for battery. The legal definition of battery arises from the statement put forward by Schloendorff which states

> *"Every human being of adult years and sound mind has a right to determine what shall be done to his own body. Any interference to a patient's body without their consent commits an assault."*

In this situation, a patient does not need to prove that they have suffered from any harm as a result of the intervention for damages to be awarded. In order for a patient to make a correct choice as to whether or not to accept treatment or to undergo a diagnostic test, they need precise information about the nature of the treatment, its benefits and risks, as well as realistic information about alternative treatments. If doctors do not give patients certain relevant information prior to obtaining consent from the patient, they will be negligent in terms of misinformation.

Information that should be made available to patients

For any given procedure, treatment or operation, the doctor needs to explain the nature of the procedure. For example, if a patient needs to have a carcinomatous growth removed from her breast, she must understand that the operation will involve an incision to her chest wall and removal of that breast, as well as a possible removal of lymph nodes in the axillary region.

The doctor must exercise sensitivity to the patient's fears that their body will undergo significant changes with such surgery, and must make available all possible treatments for a growth in the breast such as chemotherapy, and advise the patient of the prognostic outcomes following each type of therapy available. It is a legal requirement to inform the patient of risks, benefits and alternative treatments which demonstrate both good practice and the avoidance of negligence.

Doctors are often faced with litigation when patients understand the benefits of their treatment but do not understand the risks of the procedures that they are undergoing. This duty of the doctor to provide this information frankly to the patient is paramount so that the patient is furnished with all necessary information prior to making a choice.

Fortunately, many of the theories and the laws that have been passed in this area arise from known and much-publicised cases. The Bolan test suggests that a doctor is not negligent if he has acted in accordance with the practice accepted as proper by a responsible body of medical men skilled in that particular art. It is the duty of the doctor to inform the patient of all risks, even if the possibility of the risk is less than

1%, and this information should be documented in the patient's notes. It should also be documented in the consent form that the patient has signed if it is to legally cover the doctor in court.

Most patients make it clear that they would wish to be well informed about the risks of clinical procedures, and from the ethical point of view the issue is more about how best to inform, rather than whether to inform the patient. If the patient asks for particular information, then it is the doctor's duty to inform the patient of all possibilities.

This is a difficult task in medical practice, where at one end of the spectrum the doctor will want to do what is best in the interests of his patient, although this may not be evident should that patient fall victim to a less than 1% chance complication as a result of the procedure or investigation. Many doctors argue that because touching a patient without consent can constitute battery, the patient's consent is needed even when taking his pulse or examining a rash on the skin. Doctors often see patients in limited clinic times and seldom obtain specific consent for such routine parts of medical examination. Would this imply that patients could successfully sue the doctor for undertaking a routine examination which would enable the doctor to make formal clinical decisions about the patient's health ? Courts, however, do recognise the concept of "implied consent". The doctor says "I would like to measure your blood pressure", and the patient offers his arm and sits quietly while the doctor measures the blood pressure, the patient's consent is taken to be implied by his behaviour. If a competent patient refuses, then it would constitute battery if the doctor ignored this and attempted to take a blood pressure reading, despite clear communication from the patient.

In the past, many doctors have argued that the fact that a patient comes to see the doctor or is admitted to hospital does imply consent for examination. This is not the case. A competent patient could readily come to see the doctor and refuse consent to be touched in any way.

The use of consent forms
At present in medical practice, consent forms are generally used if the patient is going to be exposed to any invasive procedure. After providing the patient with adequate information about the procedure, as well as risks and benefits, doctors should document what has been said on the consent form. The patient then reads the consent form with the doctor and signs accordingly. The consent form provides a mechanism to ensure that consent is obtained, and also to communicate that fact to other members of the healthcare team.

Consent forms are not, themselves, absolute proof that valid consent was obtained to the treatment specified on the form. Most consent claims are based on failure to warn cases, with the claimant arguing that he would not have consented to the treatment if the full facts had been explained. Advice to doctors is that whenever a patient is counselled prior to a procedure, the pros and cons should be discussed as to the proposed treatment and available alternatives, and the patient's questions should be answered fully. It is useful to make a note of the main areas discussed.

Competence (capacity)
Competence has both medical and legal interpretations. For doctors, competence means the ability of patients to understand and take decisions upon any aspect of their healthcare.

A competent person must give fully informed consent before any medical procedure is undertaken. Refusal to accept *treatment* that the doctor considers to be necessary does not imply any lack of competence. In emergency, the doctor may still act (without consent) providing that it is in the best interest of the patient.

The law defines competence in children by chronological age. Exceptions arise with age, particularly in subjects under 18 years of age. Furthermore, a patient with severe dementia is unlikely to be competent to give or refuse consent for a life-saving or life-improving procedure. In medical law regarding consent, the main issues are whether the patient has capacity to give or refuse consent.

Current laws on consent

For a competent adult patient (aged over 18 years), the patient may refuse any, even life-saving treatment. Any invasion of this patient's wishes would constitute as battery in a court of law. Patients should be given information as to the nature of the procedure, and if they have been misinformed, this will also constitute battery. The doctor should also explain all common and rare serious side effects, benefits and reasonable alternatives to the treatment recommended to avoid litigation for negligence. If the patient is incompetent, then it is the doctor's duty to act in the best interests of the patient. This requires both professional judgment which relies on the Bolan test regarding a responsible body of sound medical opinion.

Whilst relatives and friends may be sources of information when judging best interests, they are not in a legal position to either give or withhold consent. In English law, there is no proxy consent for an incompetent adult. For patients under 18 years of age, the law is more complex. One of the clearer guidelines is that a doctor should not allow a person under 18 years of age to come to any serious harm should that patient often prefer to, as a minor, and/or parents refusing consent for necessary and urgent treatment. Patients between the age of 16 and 17 years of age are governed by statute. They are presumed to have capacity to give consent to medical procedures unless the contrary is shown. If they have the capacity, then can give their consent which would be of value legally.

If the patient refuses consent, then those with parental or guardian responsibility or a court of law, can override the patient and give consent to treatment which is in the child's best interests. Patients under the age of 16 years are presumed not to have the capacity for consent unless they satisfy health professionals that they do have such a capacity.

The common law case of *Gillick v West Norfolk and Wisbech Area Health Authority and another [1985] 3 All ER* established that a child under 16 years of age who does have capacity is referred to as "Gillick competent". This type of patient can give consent for medical treatment. The precise criteria for judging Gillick competence are not clear, but do include understanding key facts and the ability to come to a reasoned decision. It is unlikely that the courts would consider children aged 13 years or under to be Gillick competent in most situations, although there is no clear legal guidance on this matter. If the patient refuses consent, then the legal system can override the patient's choice and give consent to treatment which, is again, in the child's best interests. For children who are not Gillick competent, it is the duty of the parents or guardians to generally give consent. Parents are under a legal obligation to act in the child's best interests. If parents refuse consent for a procedure that a doctor thinks is strongly in the child's best interests, the doctor should inform the courts. In an emergency, if parental consent is not forthcoming and there is insufficient time to involve the courts, the doctor will be covered if his actions are those to save the child from death or serious harm. The doctor, however, is encouraged to obtain consent even in a verbal form if the parents or guardians are unable to be at the hospital at the time when a rapid decision needs to be made. A précis of the *Gillick* case is given below.

The Department of Health and Social Security issued a circular to area health authorities containing, inter alia, advice to the effect that a doctor consulted at a family planning clinic by a girl under 16 would not be acting unlawfully if he prescribed contraceptives for the girl, so long as in doing so he was acting in good faith to protect her against the harmful effects of sexual intercourse. The circular further stated that, although a doctor should proceed on the assumption that advice and treatment on contraception should not be given to a girl under 16 without parental consent and that he should try to persuade the girl to involve her parents in the matter, nevertheless the principle of confidentiality between doctor and patient applied to a girl under 16 seeking contraceptives and therefore, in exceptional cases, the doctor could prescribe contraceptives without consulting the girl's parents or obtaining their consent if in the doctor's clinical judgment it was desirable to prescribe contraceptives.

The plaintiff, who had five daughters under the age of 16, sought an assurance from her local area health authority that her daughters would not be given advice and treatment on contraception without the plaintiff's prior knowledge and consent while they were under 16. When the authority refused to give such an assurance the plaintiff brought an action against the authority and the department seeking

i. as against both the department and the area health authority, a declaration that the advice contained in the circular was unlawful, because it amounted to advice to doctors to commit the offence of causing or encouraging unlawful sexual intercourse with a girl under 16, contrary to s 28(1)a of the Sexual Offences Act 1956, or the offence of being an accessory to unlawful sexual intercourse with a girl under 16, contrary to s 6(1)b of that Act, and,

ii. as against the health authority, a declaration that a doctor or other professional person employed by it in its family planning service could not give advice and treatment on contraception to any child of the plaintiff below the age of 16 without the plaintiff's consent, because to do so would be unlawful as being inconsistent with the plaintiff's parental rights.

The judge held (i) that a doctor prescribing contraceptives to a girl under 16 in accordance with the advice contained in the department's circular would not thereby be committing an offence of causing or encouraging unlawful sexual intercourse with the girl, contrary to s 28(1) of the 1956 Act, and (ii) that parent's interest in his or her child did not amount to a 'right', but was more accurately described as a responsibility or duty, and accordingly giving advice to a girl under 16 on contraception without her parents' consent was not unlawful interference with parental 'rights'. He accordingly dismissed the plaintiff's action. The plaintiff appealed to the Court of Appeal, which allowed her appeal and granted the declarations sought, on the grounds that a child under 16 could not validly consent to contraceptive treatment without her parents' consent and that therefore the circular was unlawful. The department appealed to the House of Lords against the grant of the first declaration. The area health authority did not appeal against the granting of the second declaration.

One of the judges in the initial hearing dissented, stating that having regard to the reality that a child became increasingly independent as it grew older and that parental authority dwindled correspondingly, the law did not recognise any rule of absolute parental authority until a fixed age. Instead, parental rights were recognised by the law only as long as they were needed for the protection of the child and such rights yielded to the child's right to make his/her own decisions when he/she reached a sufficient understanding and intelligence to be capable of making up his own mind. Accordingly, a girl under 16 did not, merely by reason of her age, lack legal capacity to consent to contraceptive advice and treatment by a doctor.

Advance directives

A person can anticipate losing the mental capacity to decide or communicate how she wishes to be treated by drawing up a formal advance statement of her *values* and preferences or by naming a person who can be consulted. It will increasingly be unwise to ignore these directives, and they can be helpful to clinicians. There can be difficulties in interpreting an advance statement which is drawn up either in too general or too specific terms, and requests for illegal or clinically inappropriate treatment cannot be complied with. However, a competent adult's advance refusal of either a specific treatment (e.g. a Jehovah's Witness) has legal force.

These are statements usually written and formally witnessed made by a person when they are fully competent about the medical care he/she does or does not want to receive should they become incompetent in the future and require medical care. Whilst this is growing practice in the United States, in the United Kingdom few people have completed an advance directive. A number of cases show that competent persons can refuse specific procedures in the future if they become incompetent, and a doctor who gives such treatment in the fact of an advance directive might be liable for battery. However, it might be unwise to allow the patient to come to significant harm through following an advance directive, unless the doctor is sure that the patient's refusal was made competently and was based on all relevant information, and that the patient had considered the clinical situation which had arisen.

5.3 Confidentiality

"Whatever … I see or hear in the life of men, which ought not to be spoken of abroad, I will not divulge, as reckoning that all such should be a secret."
- from the Hippocratic Oath.

"I will respect the secrets which are confided in me, even after the patient has died."
– the Declaration of Geneva.

Confidentiality forms the core of any doctor/patient relationship. It is based upon the central ethical pillar of clinical practice among health care professionals. The fundamental concept of medical confidentiality is the view that the information the doctor learns about a patient belongs to that patient, and that the patient has a right to determine who has access to such information.

From a patient's point of view, the information given to the doctor forms the basis of trust. The doctor guarantees confidentiality to the patient in exchange for the confidence and honesty of the patient. Confidentiality supports the principle of respect for patient autonomy, a principle that emphasises the patient's right to have control over his own life.

Doctors may be given information by their patients solely because the patient believes there is an understanding that what he says will be kept confidential. If the doctor subsequently breaches that confidentiality, the patient may feel that the doctor has broken an implied promise. Breaching such confidences always has untoward consequences, particularly for the doctor/patient relationship. If the patient discovers the breach, he may lose trust in that particular doctor, or in doctors in general, resulting in his receiving less effective health care. If his complaint of confidentiality becomes widely known, this may undermine the attitude of many people towards the medical profession, with the consequences of general loss of trust and a deleterious effect on health care.

Confidentiality is an important legal as well as ethical principle. The basic rule is that the information obtain in professional confidence should be divulged only with the consent of the individual concerned. However, the rule is not absolute, and there are some common exceptions.

Legal aspects of confidentiality

There is a general legal obligation for doctors to keep what patients tell them confidential. This obligation of confidentiality is best seen as a public and not a private interest. In the legal perspective, it is in the public interest for patients to be able to trust their doctors to maintain confidentiality. For this reason, this obligation is not absolute.

There are situations in which the law obliges doctor to breach confidentiality, and situations in which the law allows doctors to breach it. In both these situations, it is important that the doctor breaches confidentiality only to the relevant person or authority. The issue of when it is lawful, and when it is not lawful, for a doctor to breach confidentiality is often a question of balancing public interests, and not of balancing private and public interests.

The General Medical Council provides professional guidelines on the issue of confidentiality for practising doctors. Whilst these do not have the force of the law, they are taken seriously by the courts where breach of confidentiality has occurred when a patient gives consent, or when the patient cannot be identified. Sharing information about a patient with other members of the healthcare team, and for the purpose of providing the best treatment, is not generally viewed by the law as a breach of confidentiality. Doctors must take reasonable precautions, however, to prevent confidential information falling into the wrong hands by ensuring that all confidential medical information is kept reasonably secure.

Obligation for doctors to breach medical confidentiality

Information must be disclosed when there is a statutory duty (i.e. one laid down in legislation). Examples of this include:
- Notification of an infectious disease – notifiable diseases (Public Health Control of Diseases Act 1984)
- Drug addiction (Misuse of Drugs Act 1973)
- Termination of pregnancy (Abortion Act 1967)
- Births and Deaths (Births and Deaths Registration Act 1953)
- Identification of patient undergoing in vitro fertility treatment with donated gametes (and the outcome of such treatment) – The Human Fertilisation and Embryology Act 1990
- Identification of donors and recipients for transplanted organs – Human Organ Transplants Act 1989
- Prevention, apprehension or prosecution of terrorists connected with Northern Ireland – Prevention of Terrorism Act 1989
- Police on request – name and address (but not clinical details) of driver of vehicle who is alleged to be guilty of an offence under the Road Traffic Act 1988
- Under Court Orders or after the provision of a Search Warrant signed by a Circuit Judge.

If a court requires the use of disclosed confidential information, failure to do so may amount to contempt, punishable by imprisonment or a fine, or both. Doctors served with a formal Court Order should comply with it, but the mere threat of being served with a Court Order is insufficient grounds to justify disclosure of information. The above laws also reflect that disclosure is permissible when required in the public interest.

On a day to day basis in medical practice, this would consist of the sharing of information with other members of the healthcare team in the interests of the patient's care. However, other situations arise when the patient's condition or activities may have serious implications on other non-suspecting members of the public. A common problem seen in this area are patients who are not medically fit to drive, and the GMS now advises doctors to inform the DVI medical officer in such circumstances. Other situations may arise when a third party is at significant risk of harm as a result of a patient's illness (e.g. the partner of an HIV positive person).

The key areas where doctors must not breach confidentiality at any cost consist of casual breaches to either satisfy another person's curiosity, provide amusement, by failure to make anonymous details in reports or publications. Furthermore, a doctor cannot disclose details of drug dependence of patients to prevent minor crime, or to help conviction in minor crime cases (most cases against property are probably considered minor crimes in this context).

Doctors must also not breach confidentiality to prevent minor harm to another individual. With regard to doctors working in the speciality of genito-urinary medicine, no information that might identify a patient examined or treated for any sexually transmitted disease should be provided to a third party, except for in a few specific situations where that third party may be in a situation of contracting a life-threatening disease, such as HIV infection. Furthermore, doctors should not write reports or disclose any confidential information which may be requested by insurance companies or employers without patients' prior written consent.

During a medical examination, either for insurance or fitness to work, it must be clear at the outset that the patient is aware of the purpose of the assessment, of the obligation that the doctor has towards third parties concerned, and that this may necessitate disclosure of personal information. Prior written consent should be obtained before such an assessment is made. Even after a patient has died, the obligation to keep the information confidential remains. If an insurance company seeks information about a deceased patient to decide whether or not to make a payment under a life assurance policy, information should not be released without the prior consent of the patient's executor, or a close relative, without being fully informed of the consequences of disclosure.

Confidentiality and access to medical records

It is often essential to pass confidential medical information about a patient between members of a healthcare team in order to provide and improve the quality of care given to the patient. In such a situation, the patient's explicit consent may not be required. Explicit consent is not needed when a medical practitioner discloses relevant information to a medical secretary to have a referral letter typed in order to request that the patient is seen by an appropriate medical specialist. Furthermore, doctors need to make relevant information available to other medical staff such as radiologists when requesting x-rays in order to establish a diagnosis. If a patient does not wish particular information to be shared with other members of the team, that wish must normally be respected. Prior to the Administration of Justice Act 1970, it was impossible to insist that medical records on a patient were made available prior to a trial. This often led to unnecessary delays in the legal case. Although it was initially intended that medical notes and records should be made available to a named medical advisor, a decision made on the grounds that laymen could not understand medical notes, or that they may find them distressing or embarrassing.

The issue of access to medical records required in connection with legal proceedings has now been largely resolved. Pre-trial disclosure is the norm in most cases. This is particularly helpful in alleged medical negligence cases or when there is a possibility of an out of court settlement. The Access to Health Records Act 1990 gives patients the right to be shown their medical records and obtain copies of these records. If the notes made are illegible or unintelligible, a patient is also within his rights to request that the records be explained. This law however only applies to medical records made after 1st November 1991. Records made prior to this date are only made available in chronic conditions, yet preliminary records are necessary to understand actions taken during the length of the illness. However, a doctor may deny a patient access to the notes if it is believed that serious harm may occur to the patient's physical or mental health as a result of seeing the records. This may be thought of as necessary in cases of intersex where genetic males present phenotypically as females at birth and are reared as females because their sexual characteristics confer to female sexual characteristics. Patients of this nature would have to deal with problems such as infertility and may have already established a successful relationship with a phenotypically normal genetic male, and such information being available could cause much unnecessary serious harm to the patient's mental health.

Furthermore, in some instances of medical practice a situation may have arisen when information was provided about the patient's condition by a spouse, relative or close friend, the doctor should also ensure that confidentiality of this informant is maintained, and notes made regarding this subject should not be made available to the patient. The doctor is not obliged to tell the patient that part of the notes have been removed unless the patient asks. In order for a patient to have access to their medical records, an application should be made in writing by the patient. This would also apply to children under the age of 16 years who are competent. Application can also be made by a third party authorised by the party in writing.

This also applies to a parent or guardian of a child under 16 years provided that prior consent is obtained for the child, or if it is evident that the child is not competent to give such consent. The court may appoint persons to apply for access to medical records if the patient is not capable of managing his/her affairs. This also applies to an executor or administrator of a patient's estate if the patient has died. It is the doctor's duty to enable the patient to see the medical records, or copies of the records, within 21 days or a maximum of 40 days, if the records are over 40 days old.

The doctor is within his rights to charge a reasonable fee for copying the records, and also for the time spent explaining the records. The patient may ask for inaccurate or misleading information to be corrected and the doctor should ensure that the correction is made if the original account is inaccurate.

GMC guidelines on the principles of confidentiality

The GMC states that patients have a right to expect that doctors will not disclose any personal information which they learn during the course of their professional duties unless they give permission. Without assurance to that confidentiality, patients may be reluctant to give doctors the information they need in order to provide optimum care. For these reasons, doctors are asked to comply with the following standards. When a doctor is responsible for confidential information, it is the duty of the doctor to ensure that the information is effectively protected against improper disclosure when it is received, transmitted, stored or disposed. When patients give consent to disclosure of information about themselves, you must ensure they understand what is being disclosed, the reasons for disclosure, and the likely consequences. You must also ensure that patients are informed whenever information about them is likely to be disclosed to others involved in their healthcare, and that they have the opportunity to withhold permission. The doctor must also respect requests by patients that information should not be disclosed to third parties, except in specific circumstances, where the health or safety of others would otherwise be at serious risk.

If confidential information is disclosed, the doctor should release only as much information is necessary for that purpose. Furthermore, when information is made available to healthcare workers, they must understand that it has been given to them in confidence, which they must respect. Any doctor who decides to disclose confidential information must be prepared to explain and justify this decision.

Disclosure of information without the patient's consent

Doctors may be in a situation where they feel that it is important to disclose confidential information for the patient's own interests. If a doctor believes that the patient is a victim of neglect, physical or sexual abuse, or is unable to give or withhold consent to disclosure, it is the duty of the doctor to give information to the appropriate responsible person or agency in order to prevent further harm to the patient. In such circumstances, information may be released without the patient's consent, but only if it is considered that the patient is unable to give consent, and that disclosure is given in the patient's best medical interests.

Some patients may be incapable of giving consent to treatment because of mental incapacity, illness or immaturity. If the doctor has been unsuccessful in persuading the patient to allow an appropriate person to be involved in the consultation, and it is felt that treatment is essential in the patient's medical interests, the doctor may disclose relevant information to an appropriate person or authority.

In rarer situations, a doctor may feel that seeking consent to disclosure of confidential information would be damaging to the patient, and that the disclosure would be in the patient's medical interests, the patient may be suffering from a terminal illness and it might be evident that they might be seriously harmed by this information. In such situations, the doctor may exercise some discretion and inform the spouse or close relative without consent.

Disclosure in the interests of others

In some situations, disclosures may be necessary in the public interest, where failure to disclose information may expose the patient or others to the risk of serious harm or death. In such circumstances, the doctor is advised to disclose information promptly to an appropriate person or authority. Examples of this include a situation where a medical colleague who is also a patient is placing the patient at risk as a result of illness or another medical condition.

Another situation may arise where a surgical colleague is known to have an HIV infection. It would be the duty of the doctor to disclose information promptly to an appropriate authority.

5.4 *Negligence*

Negligence is defined as a breach of the duty of care.

One of the biggest concerns of medical practitioners today is the threat of legal action on the grounds of negligence. The annual number of medical accidents in the NHS is around 300,000. Approximately 82,000 of these arise from incidents of medical negligence. The National Audit Office in May 2000 reported that the NHS was faced with bills amounting to £3.4bn for medical negligence claims. Unfortunately, most doctors are surprisingly unaware of the basic requirements for a successful legal action.

Duties and rights

Through the developing recognition of human right demands, the tide has turned to empower the patient. This change in attitude brings with it the changing face of the doctor patient relationship. There are duties that need to be fulfilled by the doctor but these are increasingly based on the rights that have been demanded.

Negligence may be defined as failure to come up to the standard to be expected from colleagues of similar training, skills and experience. It is the doctor's duty to remain skilled, knowledgeable and competent when delivering care. A patient who is unhappy with their treatment has a right to seek compensation for medical negligence.

If we return to the *Bolam* test which still leads the medical profession legally when deciding the standards to be expected and applied to the profession, the actions of the doctor need to be shown to be equivalent to men of similar skill. For this reason, the law may have profound difficulty in establishing that a breach of duty has taken place.

A patient who wishes to succeed in a medical negligence action must prove three things:
- – The existence of a duty of care
- – Breach of that duty
- – Damage that has occurred as a consequence of the above.

Clinical negligence can be divided crudely into two areas. These are civil negligence and criminal negligence.

Civil negligence

Civil negligence is by far the more common course of action taken against a medical practitioner. A successful claimant would be awarded damages if he can show that he was owed a duty of care by the doctor or hospital concerned, and that this duty was breached, and he suffered harm as a result of that breach of duty. The court in this situation would base its decision in such cases on the balance of probabilities, which is often referred to as "the burden of proof".

Nowadays, there is rarely any argument over the existence of duty of care between the doctor and his patient. It is far more difficult to determine whether or not the care provider reached a reasonable standard and, if not, what damage, if any, was sustained from the shortfall in care. In these cases, harm suffered by the patient must be causally related to poor standards in care for compensation to be payable.

The standard of care provided by medical practitioners is judged by reference to the Bolan test. This simply states "the doctor is not guilty of negligence if acting in accordance with the practice accepted as proper by a responsible group of men skilled in that particular art."

In other words, to be defensible the doctor must be able to call upon experienced colleagues in that speciality who will testify that the doctor's management was reasonable. The question is not whether your action was right or wrong, but whether you acted reasonably. Inexperience is no defence. If you know that a particular procedure or foreseeable complications arising from that procedure requires a level of skill or expertise beyond your own, you should refer the patient to a more experienced colleague. Giving it your best shot is simply not good enough.

Similarly, when delegating duties it is incumbent upon you as the delegating doctor to ensure that the person, whether medical or non-medical, to whom the task is delegated possesses the necessary qualifications, skills and experience to carry out the procedure to a reasonable standard. The development of protocols and guidelines may reflect a consensus view of best management of particular conditions. Failure to follow that guidance may not in itself be negligent, but is likely to mean you now have to justify by reference to a responsible body of medical opinion why management has varied an individual case. Compensation awards for damages are designed to restore the patient insofar as money is concerned, so they would be in a similar position had negligence not occurred.

Damages are divided into general damages for pain, suffering, and loss of amenity, and special damages to compensate for loss of earnings and special needs, including such things as adaptations to the home, specially adapted cars, employment of staff and private remedial therapy. Compensation payments are not made on the basis of the seriousness of the mistake but on the impact of the negligence on the patient's life.

Criminal negligence:
Some acts of medical negligence resulting in death are deemed to be so reckless that they warrant criminal prosecution. Unfortunately, there is no clear cut definition of the degree of negligence that warrants criminal prosecution. The law relies on the rather circular arrangement that cases to be prosecuted are those of a doctor's conduct which are sufficiently serious to warrant prosecution. The essence here is do demonstrate criminal behaviour. In such a case, the burden of proof is beyond reasonable doubt.

Certain acts and omissions may be criminal at one time but not another. The primary characteristics of criminal acts is that they are generally considered a public wrong as well as a moral wrong. Touching a patient inappropriately in a sexual manner is an example of this.

Criminal proceedings differ from civil proceedings in that they result in the imposition of punishment accompanied by the judgement of community condemnation.

Criminological theory is traditionally influenced by two contrasting concepts:
- Classicism: This concept emphasises free will and portrays crimes as a result of voluntary actions which have been based upon rational calculation.
- Positivism: Portrays crime as a behaviour into which the individual has been propelled by factors beyond his control such as psychiatric illness. In this situation a rehabilitative sentence might be considered to be more appropriate that imprisonment.

5.5 *Resuscitation and Euthanasia*

DNR or Do Not Resuscitate orders are instructions that a patient should not receive cardiopulmonary resuscitation (CPR) in the event that she suffers a cardiac arrest, usually in hospital.

This is an example of withholding treatment

There are few areas in medical ethics that can raise such strong and diverse views as those concerned with end of life decisions. Indeed, topics such as euthanasia, do not resuscitate orders, and even advance directives (living wills) are all too often discussed with great passion at national debates.

Within the medical profession, there is concern about the distinctions, in both practice and in theory, between easing and hastening death. As members of the public, there are numerous and conflicting concerns which range from fear that doctors may not try hard enough to save a patient's life and indeed choose to allow them to die at one end of the spectrum, whilst at the other end of the spectrum, there is concern that doctors may try too hard to keep a dying patient alive, even against his will.

In dealing with these problems, two important distinctions need to be made. These distinctions are between letting someone die versus killing them. If a doctor kills a patient, the doctor causes the patient's death. If a doctor allows a patient to die, he does not cause the patient's death – the patient's death is as a result of an illness. Philosophically, there is a clear difference between these situations. The questions that need to be answered are those of a moral code. First of all, is there any distinction between killing and allowing to die when considering the relative moral standing of withholding and withdrawing treatment from a dying patient.

These actions would hasten the death of a patient and many would argue that the doctor's actions have in fact caused that death. On an emotional level, in many situations doctors and relatives of patients who are being actively treated may realise that the patient is not benefiting or improving from the course of treatment, but rather than withdraw, the treatment is prolonged. It is, however, very difficult to make a decision regarding withdrawing treatment once it has been started. The British Medical Association states that although emotionally it may be easier to withhold treatment than to withdraw that which has been started, there are no legal or necessary moral relevant differences between the two actions. Ideally, all patients are entitled to life-saving treatment despite beliefs from the outset that these treatments will not benefit the patient. In many cases, such treatment is advocated as a trial to clarify prognosis when it is predicted that continuing treatment will not be in the best interests of the patient.

The doctrine of double effect

The principle of double effect permits an act which is foreseen to have both good and bad effects. Provided that the act is good or at least indifferent, the good effect is the reason for acting, the good effect is not caused by the bad effect. A proportionate reason exists for causing the bad effect, e.g. morphine for pain may shorten life.

The principle of the double effect permits an act which is foreseen have both good and bad effects. Provided that the act itself is at least good or indifferent; the good effect is the reason for acting; The good effect is not caused by the bad effect; A proportionate reason exists for causing the bad effect.

From a philosophical point of view, it is important to make a distinction between harms that are intended and harms that are foreseen, but not intended. Medical practice has often seen patients dying from cancer. These patients are often given heightened dosages of opiates to relieve pain by their medical care teams who will have foreseen that these actions may shorten the patient's life by their effects on respiratory depression.

In accordance to the doctrine of double effect, though it would be morally wrong to inject the morphine into the patient's blood stream with the intent of hastening death. It would not necessarily be wrong to inject it if the foreseeable consequences of it were to hasten death if the doctor's intention was to relieve pain. In accordance with the doctrine of double effect, the following criteria need to be justified for the actions of the doctor not to be deemed wrong. The acts must be good or morally neutral and independent of its consequences. The agent must intend the good effect but not the bad effect. The bad effect can be foreseen, tolerated or permitted. The bad effect must not be the means to or the direct causal result of the good effect. The good effect must outweigh the bad effect.

Who makes end of life decisions ?

Doctors, patients and families may face the question of how actively life-sustaining treatments should be pursued. In making such decisions, there should be respect for the patient autonomy, knowledge about the limitation of the treatment and promotion of the patient's best interests. In the case of a competent patient, and promoting his/her best interests. Patients are deemed to act autonomously if they act with intent, with understanding and without controlling influences. Patients of this calibre may refuse life-prolonging treatment. The medical profession needs to address these situations – would this person have refused treatment in this situation, based on her values, if she knew all the relevant facts ? If the answer is yes, then there is a reason to limit life-prolonging treatment.

If the desires were regarding treatment, then it needs to be clear whether the decision was formed with an adequate understanding of alternatives and their consequences, and that these decisions were made when the person was competent, formed without coercion or undue influence. If the person was not thought to be competent, or was influenced in making those decisions, then there is no reason to limit life-prolonging treatment. In some situations, the opposite scenario may arise when a patient requests life-prolonging treatment which may prove harmful or futile. If the patient has made this decision, having been fully advised, there is no reason not to satisfy the request.

Euthanasia

The name "euthanasia" comes from the Greek. "Eu- thanatos", which means "a good or easy death". In medical practice, this concept has been promoted in the field of palliative care to ensure a comfortable death free from pain and distress. In the late 19th century this term acquired the meaning of killing someone for their own benefit. Despite three debates over legalisation of euthanasia in the House of Lords, in the United Kingdom this activity remains illegal. Arguments concerning euthanasia are often hampered by misunderstanding or lack of clarity over terminology.
The following terminology applies:-
- Euthanasia: where X intentionally kills Y for Y's benefit.
- Active euthanasia: X performs an action which itself results in Y's death.

- Passive euthanasia: X allows Y to die by withholding or withdrawing life-prolonging treatment.
- Voluntary euthanasia: Y requests death. Y is a competent adult who wants to die.
- Non-voluntary euthanasia: Y has not expressed a preference i.e. Y is severely disabled or new-born.
- Involuntary euthanasia: death is against Y's wishes.
- Suicide: Y intentionally kills himself.
- Assisted suicide: X intentionally helps Y kill himself.
- Murder: X intentionally kills Y and for this latter reason, euthanasia remains illegal in the United Kingdom.

It must be remembered now that suicide is an accepted action by a subject and is no longer illegal. Some suicides are rational. However, those who are most disabled are unable to take their own life without assistance. Withdrawing life-prolonging treatment, which is effectively passive euthanasia is widely accepted and practised. Slow death after treatment is withdrawn may cause more suffering for the patient, therefore active euthanasia may be preferable. Dying people are sometimes sedated to a state of unconsciousness. This is often referred to as effective euthanasia although some have argued that this is no different from being dead.

Euthanasia can be justified appealing to the principles of mercy-beneficence and autonomy. Euthanasia is often termed mercy killing. The suffering associated with some diseases is so great that it out-weighs the benefits of continuing to live. Existing passive euthanasia practice imply, at least in incompetent patients, that decisions have been made suggesting that the patient's life is no longer worth living. If active euthanasia would result in less suffering, it is preferable to passive euthanasia in these cases. Respect for patient autonomy should include wishes for active euthanasia at least when the patient has reasonable grounds for preferring death to continuing illness.

Palliative Care obviates the need for euthanasia. One of the main arguments for euthanasia is the possibility of relief of suffering. Great advances have been made in palliative care. Many argue that this obviates the need for euthanasia which is why the subject has been discussed so frequently in the House of Lords select Committee for Medical Ethics. Those who are the most severely disabled or ill are the most vulnerable. They may be coerced or placed under pressure, particularly if they are elderly. Even if no one is pressuring the patient to choose euthanasia, he may want to die to save relatives the burden of looking after him.

Views differ as to whether euthanasia in such circumstances is highly undesirable, or a laudable example of autonomy. Active voluntary euthanasia, were it legalised, may then open the doors to non-voluntary mercy-killing of people who are not suffering from just a physical illness, such as those who have severe learning disabilities. From a public policy perspective, laws prohibiting euthanasia are needed to protect vulnerable innocents. This argument has a logical version and an empirical version. The logical version is that we are logically permitted to extend euthanasia to those who cannot consent or who are vulnerable to pressure to consent. There is however, no logical reason to progress from voluntary euthanasia to non-voluntary or involuntary euthanasia. The empirical version holds that, as a matter of psychological fact, undesirable practices will result when we loosen constraints on killing.
Current English laws for life-ending decisions fairly state that killing a patient for any reason is normally murder. Assisting suicide is a criminal offence.

Do not Resuscitate Orders

Cardiopulmonary arrest is the most crucial of all medical emergencies. Treatment has to be administered urgently and for this reason a decision must be made for all hospital patients whether resuscitation is appropriate should they suffer a cardiopulmonary arrest. An order for Do Not Resuscitate is an example of withholding treatment.

The British Medical Association, Royal College of Nurses and the United Kingdom Resuscitation Council 1999 guidelines state that it is appropriate to consider a Do Not Resuscitate (DNR) decision in the following circumstances.
1.   When Cardiopulmonary resuscitation is unlikely to be successful.
2.   Cardiopulmonary resuscitation is not in accord with the recorded sustained wishes of a patient who is mentally competent.
3.   Cardiopulmonary resuscitation is not in accord with a valid advanced directive.
4.   Resuscitation is likely to be followed by a length and quality of life would not be in the best interest of the patient.

These criteria are however not straightforward. Although establishing the probability of success is a question of medical expertise, its evaluation as futile is not. It is a value judgement. Possible definitions of futility include the following:-
1.   The likelihood of the patient regaining consciousness following resuscitation is less than 1%.
2.   The likelihood of the patient being in hospital following resuscitation is less than 10%.
3.   The patient will live only for a few weeks because of another untreatable terminal illness.

5.6 English Laws

A competent patient can refuse any, even life-saving treatment. Treatment of competent patients must be in their best interests. There is no legal duty to preserve life at all costs. The law recognises that a patient's best interests may be served by withholding treatment that would overall be burdensome or providing palliative treatment that could shorten life. However, it is illegal and potential murder for a doctor to take action with the intention of shortening life.

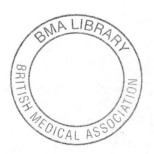

BMA LIBRARY
BRITISH MEDICAL ASSOCIATION